RECREATIVE MOVEMENT IN FURTHER EDUCATION

RECREATIVE MOVEMENT IN FURTHER EDUCATION

W. MEIER,
Senior lecturer in Movement Studies, St. Gabriel's College of Further Education, London

and M. BARANEK,
Lecturer in charge of physical education, Clarendon College of Further Education, Nottingham

MACDONALD & EVANS LTD
8 JOHN STREET, LONDON WC1N 2HY
1973

First published in September 1973

ISBN: 0 7121 1856 X

Printed in Great Britain by
Unwin Brothers Limited
The Gresham Press
Old Woking Surrey GU22 9LH

PREFACE

FURTHER education in this country takes many forms and teachers engaged in it have widely differing skills and experiences. In some instances requirements are laid down concerning the specific qualifications they must have. In other instances people start with interest, enthusiasm, some knowledge and some expertise and then proceed to equip themselves further, by attending courses, and by reading more about their subject. In the field of recreative movement there seems to have been little written for teachers of adult classes and we have received many requests to produce something of a straightforward but comprehensive nature that would meet this need.

We have taken up the challenge and tried to provide a manual of recreative movement suitable for those who are concerned with this subject in different institutions such as Colleges of Further Education, Evening Institutes, Community Centres, adult Voluntary Organisations and Youth Groups. It is intended to be suitable both for those who teach and for those who train teachers. Our justification for presuming that we have something worth offering in this field is that between us, we have had many years practical experience of training student teachers, Keep Fit leaders and trainers, students in Colleges of Further Education and leaders in the Youth Service.

Three important criteria have been behind our thinking and writing. The first is that if the material is to be of use to the practising teacher of recreative movement, it must be presented in a clear and simple manner that takes full account of practical application and it must be written in such a way that it can be understood by those whose movement knowledge is not extensive. A handbook or manual is for use, not for theoretical discussions.

Secondly, all the different aspects on which the practising

teacher needs help must be covered. For too long those who wanted material for this work have had to seek it from many sources. For example, much has been said about how important it is to study the way the body is constructed and functions and how vital it is that movement should be based on this scientific knowledge. Books on movement are usually confined to the study of the principles of movement and composition, but we have endeavoured to show, in a simple way, the relationship between the study of the body and the use of movement. In addition, we have given guidance on sources of information for extending this knowledge.

Our third criterion relates to Rudolf Laban's theories. We believe that little is written about the immediate relevance of his theories to recreative work. His writings are, and will continue to be, of immeasurable benefit to those concerned with dance and movement education. After all, Laban himself was committed to the value of recreative movement. One of his fundamental concerns was that we should understand how we use our bodies in natural activities when we work and when we play.

Some of the points we emphasise may be considered obvious and elementary and perhaps this is the very reason why they are omitted from more technical books. The simple and the obvious are frequently of fundamental importance since the skill of teaching, like most other skills, can only be acquired if it is built upon a sound, elementary base. We have therefore offered practical advice on preparation, presentation and assessment of lessons. Following from this we have given some ideas for developments and progressions. In this way we hope to encourage explorations into creative work that are based on movement activities which are meaningful to both the teacher and the students.

Until recently women have far outnumbered men in their interest in recreative movement, but we are glad to find that this situation is gradually changing and all that we have written is equally applicable to either sex.

We hope this book will help the teachers who take classes and interest the members who join them. Perhaps too, what we have written may be of value to those who give this activity their support. We have tried to underline our practical recommendations with some consideration of the fundamental principles behind this approach to recreative movement. If we have achieved some of these aims, then we shall feel we have made a useful contribution towards a fuller understanding and appreciation of an activity we believe to be of value to us all.

Acknowledgments

Our thanks are due to those who have assisted us in various ways in writing this book. We particularly wish to thank Miss Doris Jones for the diagrams, Miss Marion North for reading the script and advising us, and Miss K. Evans and Mr. W. Paul Pearson for their assistance with the anatomy and physiology section. In addition we would like to thank Mrs. Brenda Johnson and Miss Jean Clark for their help.

May 1973

WALLI MEIER
MADGE BARANEK

CONTENTS

	Page
PREFACE	v
ACKNOWLEDGMENTS	vii
LIST OF ILLUSTRATIONS	xi
INTRODUCTION	xiii
CHAPTER ONE. The class member and the teacher	1
Members and their needs	1
The teacher: qualities, skills and duties	4
CHAPTER TWO. The body—its structure and function	6
Skeletal system	6
Muscular system	14
Posture	17
Nutrition	18
Respiration	18
Circulation	19
CHAPTER THREE. Movement	22
The body as an instrument	23
Body awareness	25
Pathways	26
Rhythm	32
Relationships	35
CHAPTER FOUR. Application of movement	41
Motivation	41

Page

CHAPTER FIVE. The lesson 52
Planning 52
Progression 59
Keeping a file 63
Presentation 66
Observation and clarification 69

CHAPTER SIX. Stimuli 75
Aural 75
Tactile 80
Visual 85

APPENDIX I. Demonstrations 87
Open classes 87
Demonstrations 89

APPENDIX II.
Addresses of organisations, societies and governing bodies 92

BOOKS FOR FURTHER REFERENCE 92

BIBLIOGRAPHY 93

INDEX 95

LIST OF ILLUSTRATIONS

FIG. 1	The skeleton, with one half showing muscle groups	7
FIG. 2	The spine	9
FIG. 3	A typical vertebra	10
FIG. 4	The ankle joint and bones of the foot	11
FIG. 5	Different types of joint	12
FIG. 6	A ball and socket joint	13
FIG. 7	Ball and socket joint (shoulder)	13
FIG. 8	Knee joint	14
FIG. 9	Muscles of the upper arm showing biceps and triceps	16
FIG. 10	Postural positions; dotted lines indicate the line of gravity	17
FIG. 11	The dimensional cross	27
FIG. 11a	The octahedron	28
FIG. 12	The cube, with diagonals	29
FIG. 13	The Door plane	30
FIG. 14	The Table plane	30
FIG. 15	The Wheel plane	31
FIG. 16	The icosahedron, showing door, table and wheel planes	32
FIG. 17	The cluster	37
FIG. 18	The circle	37
FIG. 19	The line	38
FIG. 20	The triangle	38
FIG. 21	The square	39
FIG. 22	A lesson curve	52
FIG. 23	"Hotch-potch" of ideas to aid selection	57
FIG. 24	An example lesson showing the tabulation method of recording	64–5

INTRODUCTION

THERE is a danger that the ever-increasing demands made on people to-day, the many roles some of them have to play and the anxiety and frustrations of what is so often a noisy, rushed and restless existence can build up into a very unbalanced way of life. This may result in extreme tension, narrowness of outlook and general unhappiness. An urgent need for release through recreation is indicated. Recreation in its true sense is what it says, a re-creation, something made new, something that has become latent being woken up and refreshed, something urgent and exciting within us being revitalised and brought to a new enjoyment of experience and fulfilment.

Movement, which is fundamental to life, is one of the most immediate means by which this can take place. Many people are under the impression that recreative movement is just an hour's light-hearted romp, but to be wholly satisfying the session must contain a variety of ingredients which add up to a deep sense of enjoyment. Recreative movement to music as it has developed in the last few years throughout this country is aimed to provide physical and mental refreshment.

In 1929 Norah Reed, Organiser of Physical Education in Sunderland, decided to combat the demoralising effects of depression and poverty among the women around her by arranging Keep Fit classes.

This Keep Fit was based on the Swedish gymnastics used in schools at that time, adding music to the movements to give further colour and pleasure. She included working together as an important feature, in order to emphasise the companionship which she felt the women needed. The work spread to all parts of the country, did good service during the war, and in 1956 the Keep Fit Association was formed, with Norah Reed as its first President. Reflecting the changes of movement education in the country it was natural that those concerned with recreative movement should realise the value of applying Laban's principles to this work. Laban's discoveries about movement are as applicable to recreative work as they are to work study and education.

Recreative work is important in the community and in order for it to be effective it has to be presented in a way appropriate to the members. The teacher must have both experience and knowledge of the subject matter and the ability to make assessments.

In recreative movement people discover an improvement in fitness, muscle tone and general well-being. They find the companionship in an activity that is within their physical capacity and without the element of competition. Thus their confidence and sense of achievement is encouraged. The companionship offered in recreative movement lightens the feeling of isolation and leads to the sharing of problems with the comforting realisation that such problems are often not unique.

In some instances this sparks off a desire to serve the community as they become aware of situations in which they can help. Because of recreative movement's connection with music, design and colour, its members have the opportunity to widen their interests in the arts.

The exhilaration of movement and the consequent physical and mental stimulus it provides is a source of pleasure long after the class has finished. The return to everyday life brings with it a keener awareness of the participants' own individuality.

Chapter One

THE CLASS MEMBER AND THE TEACHER

Members and their needs

ANY study of recreative teaching must begin with the consideration of the class member. What is she or he like? Ages can be anything from sixteen to seventy years. Some come from very congested city areas and others from the heart of the country. Some are well-to-do, others have limited resources. There are business men, career girls and full-time housewives. There are those who lead a solitary life and those who are the centre of a big family. Temperamentally, class members can be withdrawn and reserved or gay and outgoing. This assortment of people is to be found in most groups in voluntary associations and statutory education authority classes throughout the country in such varied centres as Colleges of Further Education, community centres, clubs, church halls and village institutes. Occasionally special classes for youth groups or senior citizens, wives or business girls are arranged, but the more usual pattern is for each class to contain its own particular mixture of these. The value of recreative movement with handicapped groups is also being explored.

What are these people looking for when they join a recreative movement class? Many are concerned about their figures, they wish to slim and to be more agile. They wish to feel fit and to be rid of their aches and pains. They want not to be out of breath when they climb the stairs or to be rid of cold feet and chilblains. They wish to improve their stamina and sense of well-being. Some are looking for an opportunity to escape from the kitchen sink or the office chair, seeking a chance to be themselves, to be relieved for a time of the cares and responsibilities of life and so return home refreshed.

Many are looking for companionship, an activity to share with other men and women, linking up with the world in general and being able to use their talents working with others. Some join consciously seeking the satisfaction that comes from moving, with a wish to improve their skill, but for many it will need the teacher to bring them to the discovery of this satisfaction. These are some of the expectations which members will admit to having. The sensitive teacher may be aware of other deeper underlying needs. In any event the teacher must endeavour to be sensitive and aware, attempting to find the right blend of work which will satisfy most.

In a recreative movement class, one learns by relating to others and in so doing, each individual will be discovering his own capacities and those of others and the limitations which have to be lived with. Each class member needs to feel that it matters that he or she comes to the class, that the teacher and other members are welcoming and that the personal contributions to the group, coloured by the experiences brought from outside, are valued.

Class members vary in their ability to move, their capacity to develop and in what they think is important to learn; but the skilful teacher will use this diversity to make the lesson stimulating and flexible. Recreative movement provides the opportunity for self-fulfilment without the anxiety of competition, so prevalent to-day, particularly in physical activities, and in day-to-day living. It should be, as one member so aptly said, "a source of pleasure to draw on for the rest of the week." It is a situation in which intellectual and social class distinctions are irrelevant.

FACILITIES. A spacious, airy, light room is the first requisite. It needs to be an attractive colour and design, for although people will work with little complaint in dowdy places, they lose something of the joy and refreshment that cheerful surroundings give rise to. The floor needs to be clean, smooth, non-slip and preferably wooden, as this is warmer and less tiring to the feet than composition type surfaces. It is important that class members can make social contact with other groups in the same building, but for concentration and absorption they need privacy and quietness when working.

The overhead space should be clear of lights and other fittings, especially when small apparatus is used. Great satisfaction can be derived from a good toned and well tuned piano, providing it is skilfully played. If possible it should be on the same level as the class and positioned so that the pianist can easily see the movers. Clean, warm, spacious cloakrooms with adequate hanging space for clothes, as well as toilets and shower facilities are essential. Ideally there should be canteen facilities with comfortable seating so that members have opportunities for social contact with others. The heating should be warm enough to be welcoming, but not so warm that it saps energy. It is important to have windows that will open adequately and easily.

CLOTHING. This needs to be simple and comfortable to move in and the cut, design and colour attractive and enhancing. The materials need to be practical for laundering and travelling and of a kind that give warmth in winter, coolness in summer and present an attractive image to any audience. Multicolours and shiny designs confuse the clarity of the movement and should be avoided. Teachers should remember that leotards and catsuits are very figure-revealing and that very few women can look attractive in this form of dress. This is why many women prefer the softer line of a tunic. The tunic length and the proportions of the figure should be taken into consideration, to avoid an unflattering back view.

Footless tights give warmth in winter and improve most people's leg appearance. Cardigans blur the figure outline, while waist-length fitted jackets in the same material as the tunic give a trim look. It is recommended that movement should be done bare-foot, so that the muscles of the feet can be used freely and thus be kept supple and strong (further reference to this point is made in Chapter Two) but the teacher must be responsible for advising class members according to their needs and the conditions of the room. Very dirty, cold or splintery floors make bare-foot work unsuitable.

New members, especially heavily built ones, will need to come to bare-foot work gradually, or the arches of their feet will suffer. In these cases the teacher should recommend a non-slip foot covering which will allow maximum freedom to move. The teacher must warn members of the great danger of working in socks or tights with feet. Many sporting magazines advertise a good selection of equipment for movement. Last but not least it is worth noting that watches, jewellery and badges can cause accidents if worn when moving and certainly they spoil the "ready for action" look.

The teacher—qualities, skills and duties

QUALITIES. Do you understand and believe in the value of recreative movement? Does movement give you sufficient exhilaration and enjoyment to make you want to share it with other people? Are you able to make people enjoy working with you? Have you the physical capacity and stamina to sustain the hard work and responsibilities of teaching? Have you the ability to make decisions whilst still being able to accept other people's ideas? Can you assess the needs of both the individual and the group? Have you a sense of humour and are you a paragon of virtue?

If the answer to all the above is "yes" then you will make an excellent teacher! Obviously, it is rare that such an excellence exists in one person, but it is worth thinking about the relative importance of the different aspects of leadership. It is not each aspect in isolation that is important, but the blending of these in proportions according to the requirements of each situation. It is no good having a sense of humour if you allow it to get in the way of the main objectives. Used to flavour the lesson it releases tensions and creates warmth of atmosphere through sharing. Certainly you must work hard to plan your lessons, but do not mistake unnecessary worry for zeal.

In order to provide a class which will satisfy all the varied demands of its members, thorough preparation is needed and this involves mental and physical energy. For some teachers, this has to be done in addition to a full-time job. For this reason, teachers are urged to consider carefully the number of classes they accept. It is not the number of classes, but the quality of teaching that decides the value of a teacher.

The relationship established in the class depends greatly on personal example. It is the teacher's attitude to the class which influences the attitude of the class members one to another. Their consideration for one another reflects the teacher's consideration for them. He or she must be an example (regardless of how they may feel) in appearance and behaviour. They must be punctual to start and stop the class, but available before and after, as this will enable them to make the necessary individual contacts. It is their responsibility to see that the working conditions and equipment are satisfactory before the class arrives and left in an equally good condition at the end. Every leader should take time and trouble to make themselves pleasant to look at, to create an image worthy of the work.

SKILLS AND RESPONSIBILITIES. Teachers must have the ability to lead and guide, but not to dictate, to draw out from the class ideas and suggestions, to give opportunity for class contribution, without taking away security and confidence. They may be an authority on movement, but can they retain the interest of their classes? They need the courage to work the members to their capacity and to make full use of the special skills available in any group of people.

An intrinsic part of a teacher's responsibility is looking ahead to see the possible development of the class and help the members to see and accept it. Much of this will depend on the teacher's ability to recognise the class in its immediate setting relating to outside places, people and situations, so that these can enrich the presentation and widen the horizons. It is the teachers' responsibility to be outward looking and to be aware of other approaches which they may be able to incorporate into their work. It is important however to see that the basic objectives are not distorted by outside influences.

Chapter Two

THE BODY, ITS STRUCTURE AND FUNCTION

THERE are many comprehensive books written on anatomy and physiology and no attempt is being made here to cover this field in depth. It is however extremely important to compose movement activities with some knowledge of the machinery that is to perform them. If a movement action is to be beneficial it must be within the natural compass of the joints and muscles involved.

The structure of the human form is composed of innumerable cells, each one containing a living substance known as protoplasm. These living organisms have the power, by dividing and sub-dividing, to multiply, grow and regenerate themselves when damaged. They vary in shape and size according to the functions for which they are created and are grouped together to form tissues such as bone and muscle, and organs such as heart and liver. Combinations of these constitute systems such as respiratory, digestive or nervous systems. These systems have a remarkable ability to work as one unit. It is when this unity breaks down due to weakness or damage to one system, that the efficiency of the whole is disrupted and the person becomes ill.

Skeletal system

The skeleton is a framework made up of 206 bones and forming one fifth of the body weight. Bones are rigid, differing in size and shape according to their function, with ridges and projections for muscular attachments, as shown in Fig. 1. The broader thick bones bear weight, the curved bones enclose and protect and the long light ones allow for movement.

There are three bony masses (*see* page 8):

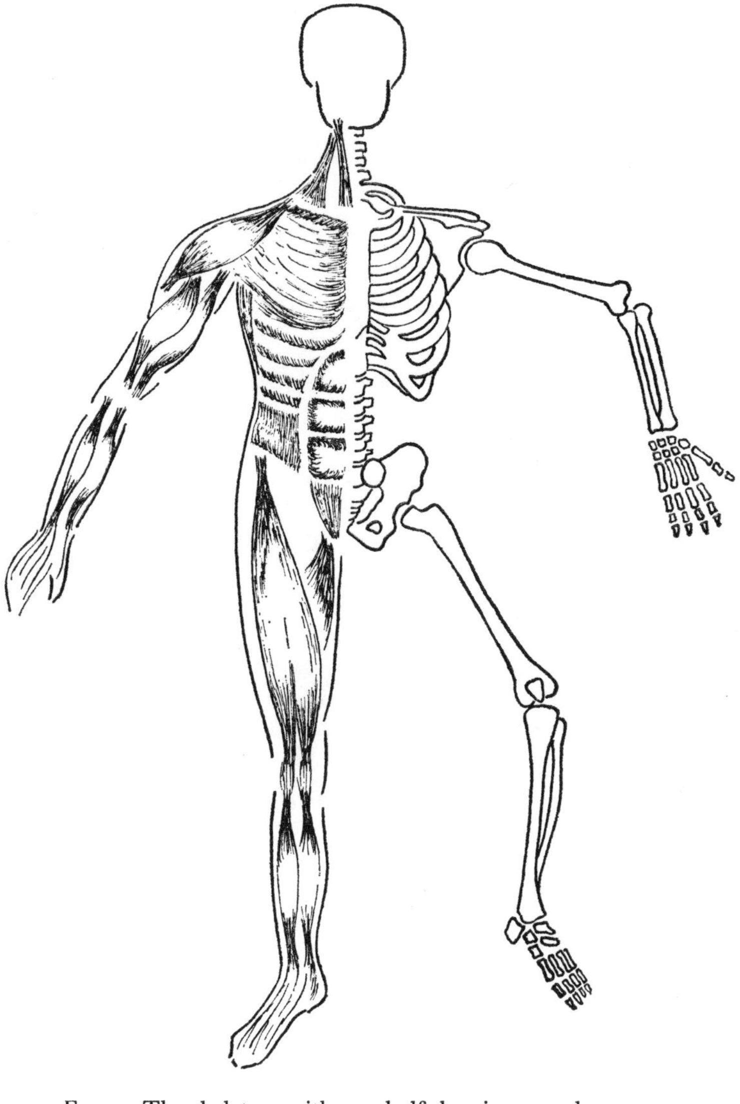

FIG. 1. The skeleton, with one half showing muscle groups

(*a*) the skull—to protect the brain;

(*b*) the thorax or chest—to protect the heart and lungs but ribbed to allow for movement;

(*c*) the abdominal cavity—basin-like to support the internal organs.

These three bony cavities are attached to the back-bone or spine, which is composed of thirty-three bones of which nine are fused. They are:

neck or cervical (7)
upper back or dorsal (12)
waist or lumbar (5)
pelvis/sacrum (5) } fused
pelvis/coccyx (4) }

Back and side views of the spine are shown in Fig. 2.

Each vertebra in the cervical, dorsal and lumbar regions has two parts; a cavity through which passes the spinal cord and three protecting wing-like structures for muscular and rib attachments. The centre projection limits the movement of the spine backwards. There is a disc of cartilage between each vertebra which serves as a shock absorber and makes the spine resilient and supple. At the top of the spine, balanced on the atlas vertebra, is the head. Attached to the dorsal vertebra are twelve pairs of ribs, which, with the sternum, form the rib cage. Attached to the sacrum are the pelvic bones. The spine has compensatory curves, concave in the neck and lumbar regions, convex in the dorsal, and it is formed in this way to facilitate movement, resilience and balance. The movements of the spine are as follows:

flexion forwards
extension
flexion sideways right and left
arch or flexion backwards (slight)
rotation with twist

These movements are evident when the spine moves as a whole as in the large body actions, but they can also be achieved in

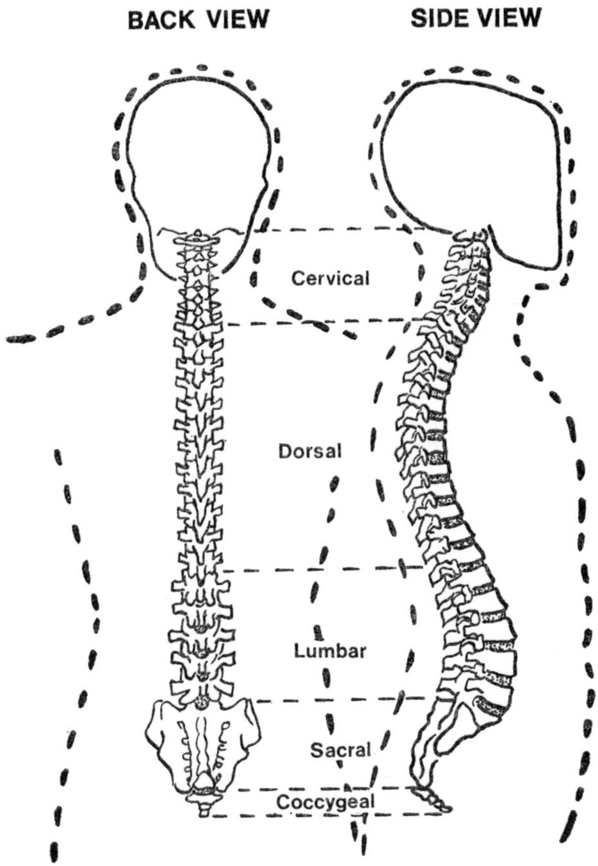

FIG. 2. The spine

the varying regions of the spine to some degree. Figure 3 shows a typical vertebra.

(*a*) *The pelvic girdle* is composed of two strong hip or pelvic bones forming the floor of the abdominal cavity. This is attached to the spine by the sacrum. This and the coccyx form the back of the cavity. The long thigh bones of the legs (femur) are attached either side of the pelvic bones. At the opposite end they meet the lower leg bones, the tibia and the fibula, which together with the patella form the knee joint. The pelvic girdle is strong, designed for weight bearing and balance.

(*b*) *The shoulder girdle* is made up of very light yoke-like bones. The collar bones (clavicles) are attached on either side

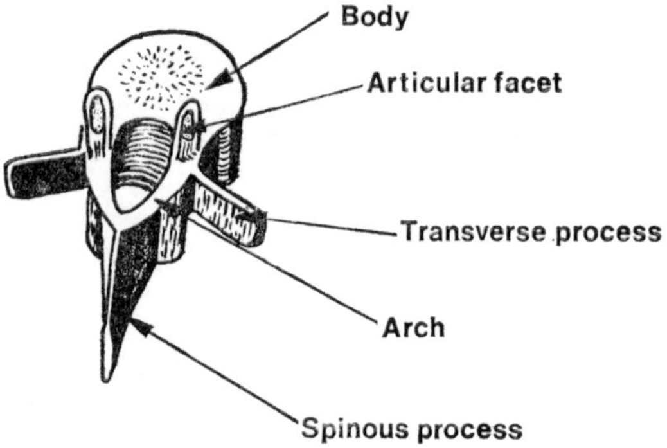

FIG. 3. A typical vertebra

of the sternum by pliable cartilages. At the back are the shoulder blades (scapulae) which have a sliding action. These come together with the head of the upper arm bone (humerus) to form a very mobile ball and socket joint. At the lower end of the humerus the radius and ulna meet to form the elbow joint.

(*c*) *Both hands and feet* are constructed in a similar manner and consist of:

feet	seven tarsal or ankle bones attached to the lower ends of the tibia and fibula.
	five metatarsal bones forming the sole of the foot.
	fourteen phlanges forming the toes (see Fig. 4).
hands	eight carpal or wrist bones attached to the lower ends of the ulna and radius.
	five metacarpal bones forming the palm of the hand.
	fourteen phlanges forming the fingers.

It is the composition of the small compact bones and their articulations together with the support of the ligaments and muscles that give strength and flexibility to the hands and feet.

The longer thinner bones of the hand together with the power of the thumb to rotate give the hand dexterity. In the foot the bending strength of the longitudinal and transverse ligaments, together with the surrounding muscles, make and retain the longitudinal and transverse arches. If these arches become flattened due to strained ligaments and muscular weakness the

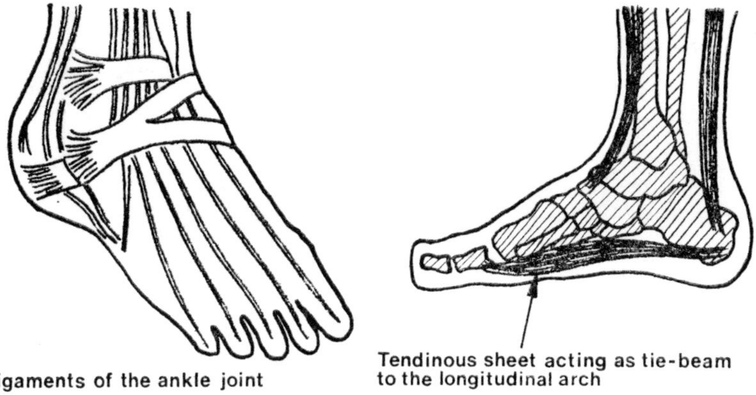

FIG. 4. The ankle joint and bones of the foot

foot is deprived of its normal spring and resilience. It is not surprising that foot troubles are common when one remembers that bones are confined within a shoe for the greater part of everyday. Circulation is restricted and the majority of the joints and muscles are unused. It is for this reason that great emphasis is placed on barefoot work and time given to warming, mobilising and strengthening the feet.

JOINTS. A joint is formed at the junction of two or sometimes three adjacent bones. The articular surfaces are covered by cartilage. They are held together by very strong, almost non-elastic tissues called ligaments. These are generally short bands together, but sometimes they are capsular. The bone surfaces within a joint are covered by a fine gauze-like tissue called synovial membrane which secretes synovial fluid to lubricate the joint and prevent friction. Some joints which bear weight or are subject to jarring have pads of resilient cartilage between the bony surfaces, for example the spine. The type and range of movement within joints varies according to the shape of the bone endings, the nearness of the bone ends

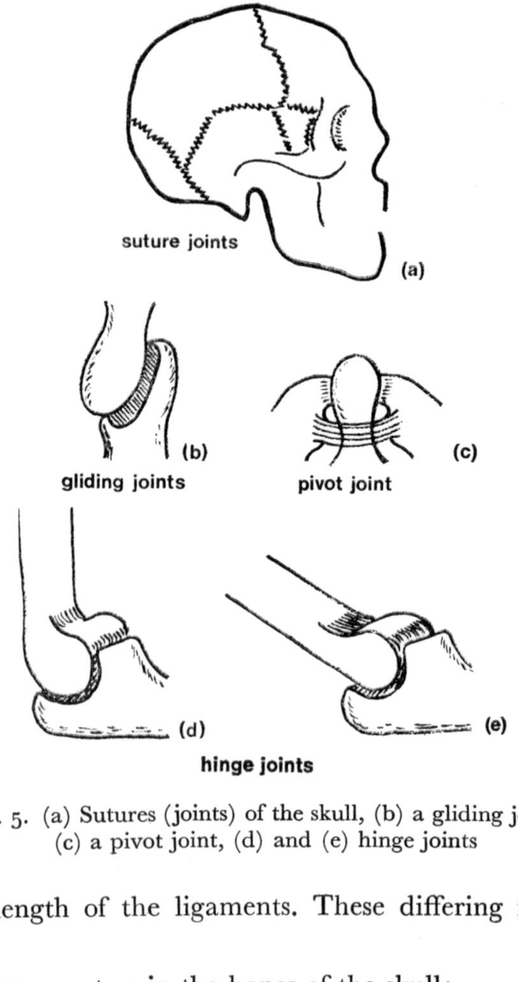

FIG. 5. (a) Sutures (joints) of the skull, (b) a gliding joint, (c) a pivot joint, (d) and (e) hinge joints

and the length of the ligaments. These differing formations allow for:

no movement as in the bones of the skull;
limited or slight movement as in the ribs;
reasonably free movement as in the shoulder.

The structure of the joint (see Fig. 5) determines its functions. The four structures are:

(*a*) ball and socket joints (see Figs. 6 and 7) *e.g.* hip and shoulder joints. These allow great freedom of movement to

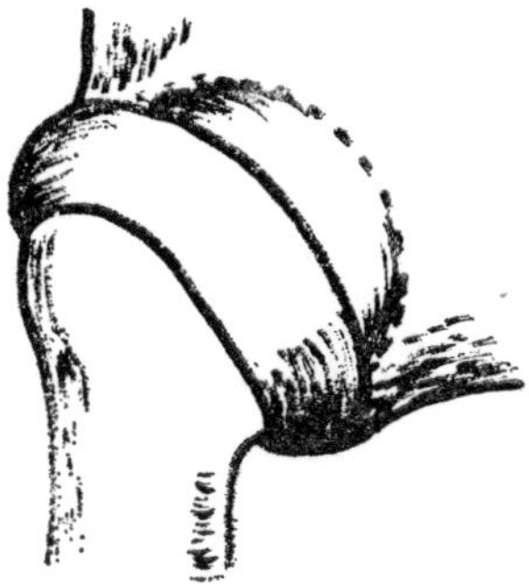

FIG. 6. A ball and socket joint (hip)

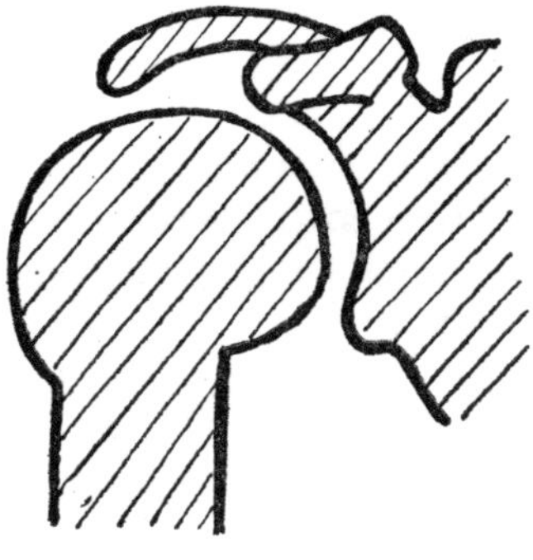

FIG. 7. Ball and socket joint (shoulder)

swing and circle the limbs—circumduction, to lift the limbs away from the body—abduction, to bring the limbs back to the body—adduction, to turn the limbs inward or outward—and rotation.

(*b*) hinge joint *e.g.* knee and elbow joints (see Fig. 8). The bone structure limits the joint to certain movements; these are extension and flexion. The ability of these joints to "lock" gives them firmness when taking weight.

(*c*) pivot joints *e.g.* radio-ulnar joint. These give a limited amount of movement, but are important as they add greatly to the versatility of the hand and arm action.

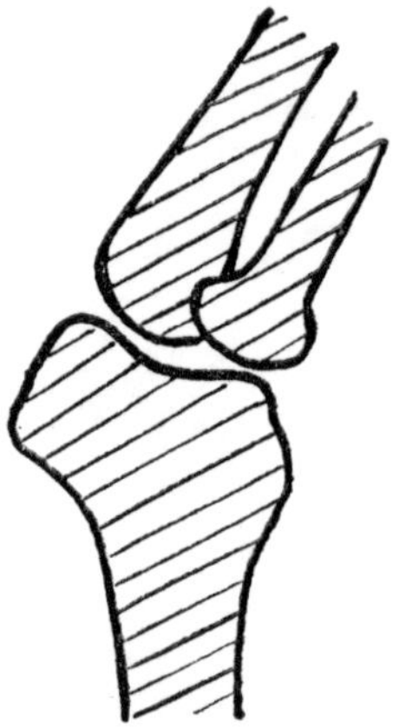

FIG. 8. Knee joint

(*d*) gliding joints *e.g.* shoulder blades or scapulae, tarsal and carpal joints. These add to the flexibility of the shoulders, ankles and wrists. The movement range is limited only by the muscles and ligaments.

The spine has not been included in any one of these groups because it is composed of a series of joints.

Muscular system

Muscle consists of elongated muscle cells or fibres which contract and relax in response to stimuli. Muscle contraction produces movement and heat. There are three types of muscle in the body:

voluntary or skeletal muscle which appears faintly striated;

involuntary or plain muscle as in the stomach, intestines, bladder and uterus;
cardiac muscle.

Skeletal muscle is made up of a large number of fibres each about 1½ in. long and as thick as a human hair. Each fibre is enclosed in an elastic sheath of connective tissue within which lie blood vessels and nerve endings. Groups of these fibres form the belly of the muscle which narrows at each end into white fibrous tissue called tendons. Each muscle has an origin and an insertion. The origin is that end of the muscle which is attached to the bone, and which normally remains static during movement. The insertion is attached to the bone which is normally pulled towards the origin. The functions of muscles are to:

cause movement;
give added support and protection to a joint or organ;
give shape and covering to the body;
produce heat.

Each muscle can only be responsible for one action, and therefore muscles need to work in opposing pairs or groups. For example, when the biceps muscle contracts the elbow bends and the opposing triceps muscle relaxes. To extend the arm, the triceps muscle must contract to pull the arm straight, and the biceps muscle must relax. Muscles can operate in two ways. These are:

static muscular action in which the muscles work in sustained tension to maintain a balance or held shape, and

dynamic muscular action in which the muscles alternate between contraction and relaxation as in locomotion or other body activities.

This alternating rhythm assists the circulation by working on the veins with a pumping action bringing the blood back to the heart. Figure 9 shows the muscles of the upper arm.

Muscle fibres are called into action by a stimulus from the brain, through the motor nerve to the muscle fibre. A chemical action is initiated, energy is released, some of which is converted into movement, through muscle contraction and the rest is utilised as body heat. As a result of this body action a waste

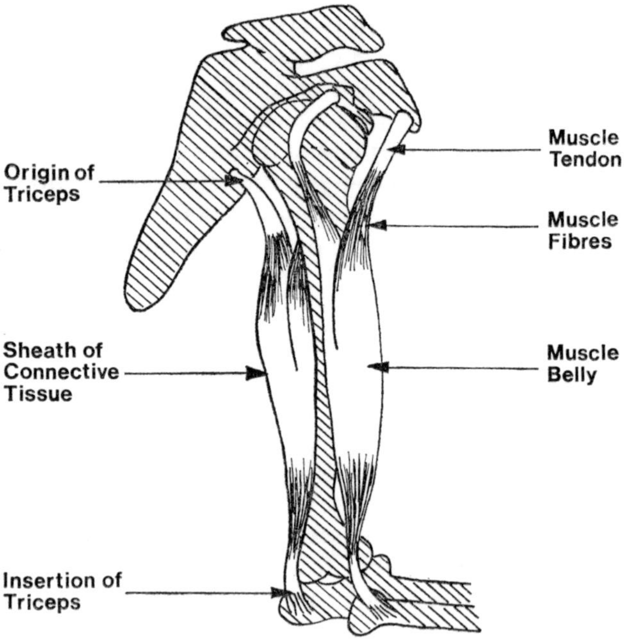

FIG. 9. Muscles of the upper arm showing biceps and triceps

product known as lactic acid is formed. When all the fibres in a muscle are fully contracted for a period of time the pressure within the muscle prevents the flow of blood, allowing the lactic acid to accumulate. This causes fatigue and pain, which can only be relieved by relaxing the muscle and allowing the flow of blood to be renewed. Stiffness in muscles after concentrated movement or from cold can be dispelled by "limbering activities."

A muscle is never completely without tension. Certain fibres are always in action, even during sleep, retaining muscle tone and keeping the body ready for a sudden call to action. This tone varies in different muscle groups; those concerned with posture retain a high degree of tension, as do those maintaining the arches of the feet. The general degree of muscle tone varies according to the health of the individual. The elasticity of muscles can "fade" due to inactivity or over-activity and it is also affected by age and nutrition.

Posture

The feet provide the base upon which the whole weight rests when standing or walking and the alignment of the body is affected by the position and condition of the feet. The side view of the body should show that the line of gravity passes from just in front of the ankle joint, through the centre of the knee, hip joint, shoulder joint and ear. In this way the body is well balanced and firmly supported from the feet upwards. Postural positions are shown in Fig. 10.

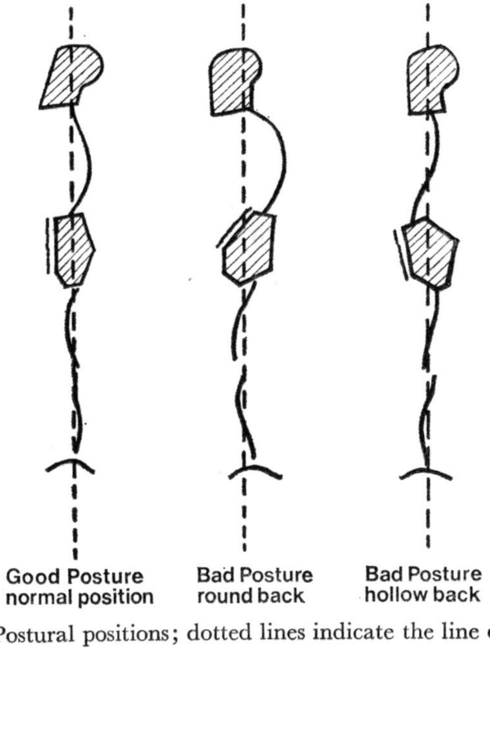

FIG. 10. Postural positions; dotted lines indicate the line of gravity

Projection of any part of the body out of this alignment involves the body in strong compensatory muscle actions and the strain on the spine and feet is increased even further if the individual is overweight. Over a period of time this will result in accumulative strain and eventually cause permanent postural defects. When the body is out of line of gravity some of the joints will be operating at a disadvantage, thus causing cartilage damage through friction.

The way in which a person carries himself is indicative of his inner feelings and state of mind; this can also work in reverse—that is, by consciously taking up good poise, the inner attitude is affected and changed.

In order to achieve this the body requires an efficient fuel service, provided by a balanced diet and fresh air, and a transport system in the form of a good supply of blood.

Nutrition

Correct nutrition is essential for maintaining the body in a healthy efficient working condition. The main food components are proteins for building and repairing tissues, carbohydrates and fats for producing energy, vitamins and mineral salts for protection against disease. Therefore it is necessary for the daily diet to contain something from each of these groups. The proportions should be matched to the physical demands, the balance between consumption and combustion always being maintained. For example, it would be unwise to omit energy-giving foods from the diet.

Slimming in this way undermines the general health. Excess energy goods can cause overweight problems, particularly for those in sedentary occupations. The digestive system is assisted by exercise which increases combustion and helps elimination of waste products. When the metabolic rate is correctly established, excess weight is avoided. Exercise also improves the muscle tone and general alignment of the body. The internal organs are held in this correct position and the figure has a slim, trim look.

Respiration

The function of respiration is to remove carbon dioxide from the blood and to replenish it with oxygen. Exercise increases the ability to make full use of the lungs so that the air intake is increased, thus improving the supply of oxygen to the blood. The improved muscle efficiency of the thoracic cage has a beneficial influence on the maintenance of posture. Lungs which are regularly filled to capacity with air have a greater resistance to disease. An insufficient supply of oxygen to the blood slows up the process of waste elimination, thus increasing the toxic content of the body, which results in a feeling of fatigue and listlessness. Room ventilation and movement resulting in increased respiration will counteract this feeling. Deep, slow rhythmic breathing has a calming effect upon the body, encourages relaxation, and, if applied consciously in moments of stress and nervous tension, gives immediate relief.

Circulation

The blood travels from the heart to every cell in the body. It is a vital transport system which delivers the food and oxygen to the cells and carries away the waste products. It distributes the hormones and the agents that fight disease as well as those that rebuild worn and damaged tissues. As exercise increases respiration, it also affects the rate of the heart beat and the volume of blood pumped round the body. Stepping up the ratio of servicing to the systems, including the brain, increases efficiency. Exercising strengthens the heart muscle so that it is capable of propulsing more blood per beat. The elastic tissue in the arteries is maintained in good condition through constant use and muscular action working on the walls of the veins assists the flow of venous blood to the heart, thus avoiding heightened blood pressure. Pain and stiffness can be relieved by maintaining an efficient circulation.

The body works best at its normal temperature of 37°C. If this falls or rises excessively the body functions are impaired. This is why temperature readings play such an important part in medical treatment. The body must have a device for regulating the amount of heat made or lost. Since heat is generated constantly it is simple to keep the body heat steady by releasing it through the mechanism of the skin. On a warm day the capillaries dilate and flush the skin with blood, thus losing heat through radiation. On a cold day these capilliaries contract, thus removing the blood from the surface so that the body heat is retained. The sweat glands release perspiration (water and salt) on to the skin where it evaporates, so causing further heat loss. To counteract this showers are taken after exercise, so that the skin is cleansed and dried before changing, so minimising the dangerous effects from continued loss of heat when damp clothing is retained.

LIFTING AND CARRYING. We are all concerned with thousands of small repetitive jobs which make very slight demands on our body's energy for a single performance, but which constantly repeated, in poor working conditions or with unsuitable action, build up what is known as cumulative strain. Tension held in a muscle restricts the flow of blood and the removal of waste so that the muscle can become shortened and under-nourished. This leads to fibrositus. The teacher of movement can help the members in her class to avoid such strain by training their awareness of the following basic methods of working:

(*a*) stepping into an action allowing free movement of the body from one foot to another, making sure that when the foot is outwardly rotated the knee joint is also in the same position. Failure to do this puts undue strain on the knee joint and the arch of the foot.

(*b*) relaxing the knees before looking down or lowering the body, thus preventing an uneven strain on the spinal discs.

(*c*) extending the spine by reaching upwards with the top of the head to straighten the neck.

(*d*) handling objects with suitable holds so that the palm or base of the fingers take the strain and the weight of the object is supported by the big muscles, as near to the body as possible.

For further information on this subject the teacher will find it useful to read *Housework with Ease* by McClurg Anderson.

FIRST AID. In spite of all precautionary planning, accidents are likely to occur in movement sessions, so it is important that the teacher is equipped to deal with the type of injuries likely to happen. First Aid study with St. John Ambulance or the Red Cross Associations would be useful. The reference section of this book recommends books on the subject.

Chapter Three

MOVEMENT

THE nature of the sort of people that we are is expressed by the unconscious movement choice we make in the necessary actions of everyday living. Imagine you are standing outside an Evening Centre and watching everyone entering the building. There are people of all shapes and sizes passing by, the tall, the short, wide, thin, round and angular. Here is one with sudden hasty movements, another entering with slow even deliberate steps, another squeezing by surreptitiously, another embracing as it were all who came in with him. Some dive through the centre of the crowd, others weave their way carefully in and out. So one can go on, seeing the many variations that indicate the personality and the feelings and attitudes uppermost at the time.

Rudolf Laban observed the movements of people at work and play in many parts of the world and it was from these observations that he became aware not only of the vast differences of build, but of the variety of gestures and qualities of movement people chose to use. He observed that it does not always follow that the large heavy man tends to move sluggishly, or a small thin person very quickly and precisely. It might well be the reverse, the large heavy man might move with very light delicate actions and the latter with strong vigorous movements.

He observed that although the physical frame in which we live influences our way of moving, it does not dictate the inner attitude or ability to control the way in which we wish to move. So a small person can experience the feeling of what it is like to be tall and strong, and a large person can experience the feeling of being thin, narrow and neat. These are only simple examples of the vast variety of builds and qualities which are observable. It was these differences which Laban studied in order to formulate his observations of human movement. He became aware that although there was such an enormous variety of movement possibilities, most people moved in a very limited and unbalanced way, not always suited to the tasks in which they were employed. His investigations centred on the possibilities of improving the relationship between the task and the movement used to perform it.

Out of this research into movement there developed the vocabulary from which all types of movement may arise, from the purely artistic creative work to the analysis of the functional mechanical actions. In education, rich movement experience coupled with the creative possibilities contributes to the natural growth and development of young people. In therapy, there is the opportunity for the re-understanding of self through body action and communication through moving with others. In recreation, all these aspects must contribute their part when we consider the full meaning of the word.

There is no such thing as one channel of movement, but rather a never-ending fountain. Unlike some schools of movement which are self-contained, the work originating from Laban's ideas is limitless; it presupposes no particular style of movement and cannot be encompassed by any one person. In order to apply Laban's theory of movement to recreative movement, we will consider each aspect in turn:

the body as an instrument;
pathways;
rhythm;
relationship.

The body as an instrument

Everyday actions whether in the home, factory, office, shop or street involve the body in the actions of bending, stretching or twisting. These are the basic mechanical actions which, when combined, produce our main body activities and govern every aspect of living. These main body activities are:

(*a*) gesture;

(*b*) weight transference and locomotion, including stepping;
(*c*) elevation, including jumping;
(*d*) turns;
(*e*) stillness.

(*a*) *Gesture* is a movement which does not support the weight of the body. Gesturing movements are all those of gathering in and scattering out and creating patterns in the air. These movements can be performed with legs and other body parts, as well as with the arms.

(*b*) *Weight transference* means moving the body weight from one point of support to another. This can occur on the spot as when going from standing to kneeling to sitting, or in rocking or lilting actions. Weight transference can lead into locomotion by weight being taken on different parts of the body, leading to travelling such as creeping and crawling, but more usually on the legs where the weight sliding and rolling is transferred from one foot to another, so producing walking, running, leaping, galloping—in fact all variations of stepping.

(*c*) *Elevation, including jumping*. Elevation is the lifting away from the ground resisting the pull of gravity. This can be achieved with the whole or parts of the body. A strong sudden movement of the legs or hips will eject the body into the air, giving a jump. There are five basic take-offs or jumps and they are:

one foot to the other;
one foot to the same foot;
one foot to two feet;
two feet to one foot;
two feet to two feet.

(*d*) *Turns*. Turning leads the body to have a change of front and therefore a changed view of the room and other people. A number of turns are possible by changing the body emphasis, *e.g.*

body opening will give open turn;
body closing will give closed turn;

body within line of gravity stable (balanced) turn;
body out of line of gravity a labile (off balance) turn.

Turns are possible on a variety of supports such as hips, knees, shoulders. If one part of the body is moved in opposition to another part when turning, a twisting action occurs. It is the element of resistance which is important.

(*e*) *Stillness.* This is as much an action as any other movement, particularly if held in a difficult position. It requires control and balance of tensions in order to maintain the body position. There are three types of stillness:

(1) where the body is completely relaxed;
(2) where there is a definite stop with a sense of arrival;
(3) a more subtle stopping whereby the flow of movement is suspended temporarily.

So far only the basic activities have been considered, but within these, if a greater stress is laid on body awareness, clarity will be improved and wider variations will be available.

Body Awareness

(*a*) *Symmetry and asymmetry.* When both sides of the body work together a stable, balanced situation is created. This is symmetrical. When one side of the body is stressed, the movement may become off-balance and lead to travelling and turning. This is asymmetrical.

(*b*) *Focus on body parts.* There can be an emphasis on different parts of the body, not only in a supporting or balancing role, but where they play a definite part in making gestures or interesting patterns. This could happen with the focus jumping from part to part such as hands to knees, shoulders to heels. Alternatively, parts can be used with emphasis on their coming together and withdrawing, or actually making contact as in clapping or clicking heels. Parts of the body may also lead a movement. An elbow, the edge of a hand, thumb or finger, the outside surface of the leg or the surfaces of the trunk may lead, giving movements of very varied character.

(*c*) *The flow of movement* can be observed passing through the body in a successive or simultaneous movement. In a successive movement the flow passes from one joint to another, sometimes through neighbouring joints consecutively as in hip, knee, ankle, toe or through a more unusual route through left knee, right shoulder, left elbow, head, right leg.

In simultaneous movement all parts of the body are equally involved throughout the action. The flow of movement may pass from the centre of the body outwards and conversely from the periphery to the centre.

(*d*) *Body shape.* As soon as the flow of movement is held the body creates a definite shape in space. This shape varies according to the movement which has preceded it. These fall into four main categories. Rounded, curving movements will result in a curved body shape, stretching outward movements in a broad shape, elongated movements in an arrow-like shape and twisting movements in a screw-like shape. It must be remembered that the creating of shapes can occur in parts as well as the whole and in motion as well as stillness.

Combinations of the body activities using the natural order of preparation, action, and recovery are called movement phrases.

It is useful to consider this section on "the body as an instrument" as dealing with the part of the movement that answers the question "What is the body doing?" *e.g.* is the activity travelling or turning? What part of the body is leading? Is the body action symmetric or asymmetric, successive or simultaneous?

Pathways

The body can move into the surrounding areas of space in different ways:

(*a*) *Away and towards the body.* These are movements that radiate from the centre of the body to the periphery and return in a spoke-like way.

(*b*) *Around the body.* Here the movement encircles the body.

(*c*) *Near and far.* Movements can occur at different degrees of distance from the centre of the body which will affect the size of the movement.

(*d*) *At varying levels.* High—referring to space above the shoulders. Medium—referring to space around the waist level. Deep—referring to the space below the hips.

(*e*) *Air and floor patterns.* Movements of the body create different patterns in the air by gesture and shaping and on the floor with stepping, or other forms of locomotion. The four basic patterns that arise are straight lines, angular, curved and twisted shapes. An angular pattern is created by two straight consecutive lines with an immediate change of direction. A twisted shape is created by two consecutive curves with a gradual change of direction.

(*f*) *Directions.* It is important to distinguish between personal space and general space. Personal space relates to the individual mover and in this context the direction forward would always be in relation to the front of the body, regardless of the direction faced. General space relates to parts of the room. Orientation is made from outside points, *e.g.* piano, door, wall or window.

SPACE FORMS

(*a*) *Dimensional Cross* (Fig. 11). There are six fundamental

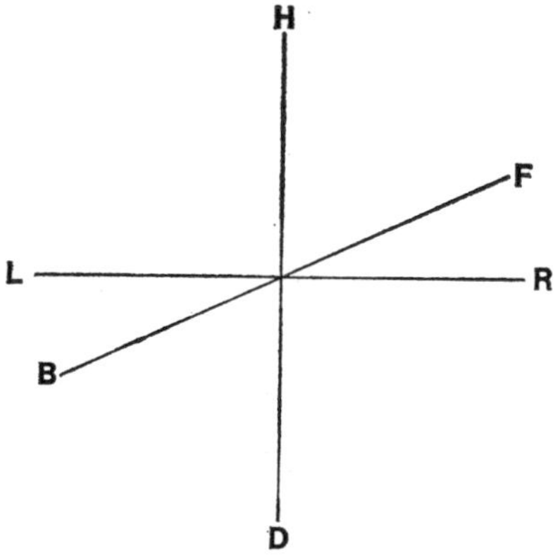

FIG. 11. The dimensional cross

directions from the centre of the body which result from the following body actions and form a dimensional cross.
These are:

rising leads to high;
sinking leads to deep;
opening leads to left or right;
closing leads to left or right;
advancing leads to forwards;
retreating leads to backwards.

Moving in these six fundamental directions gives a feeling of stability and balance as the body retains its position with the line of gravity. Moving around the circumference of these six points shapes an octahedron, as in Fig. 11 (a).

(*b*) *Diagonal cross.* Diagonal directions from the centre of the

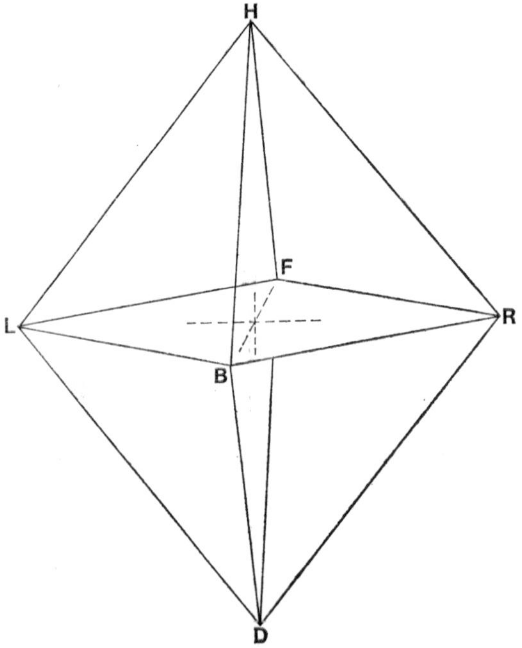

FIG. 11a. The octahedron

body are arrived at by combining three bodily activities. Using the right side:

rising, opening and advancing leads to high right forward;
sinking, closing and retreating leads to deep left back;
sinking, opening and retreating leads to deep right back;
rising, closing and advancing leads to high left forwards;
rising, closing and retreating leads to high left back;
sinking, opening and advancing leads to deep right forwards;
rising, opening and retreating leads to high right back;
sinking, closing and advancing leads to deep left forwards.

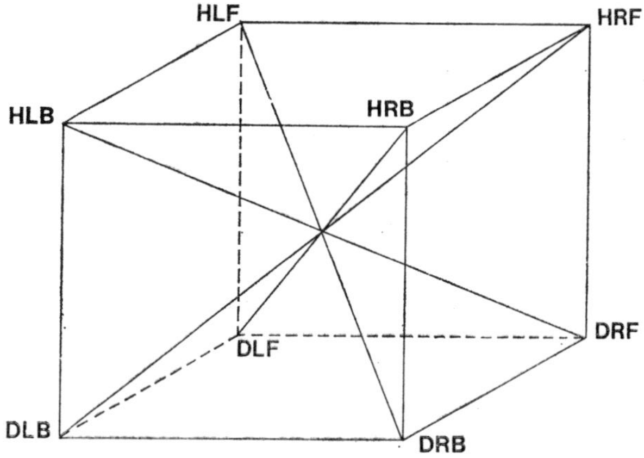

FIG. 12. The cube, with diagonals

Moving into these diagonal directions causes the body to move out of the line of gravity and a feeling of instability and unbalance is caused. Moving around the circumference of these eight points of orientation gives a cube (see Fig. 12).

(*c*) *Planes of movement.* Twelve other directions from the centre of the body are created by combining two activities, using the right side these are:

rising while opening leads to high right;
sinking while closing leads to deep left;

rising while closing leads to high left;
sinking while opening leads to deep right.
The pathway linking these four points of orientation peripherally is known as the Door Plane (Fig. 13).

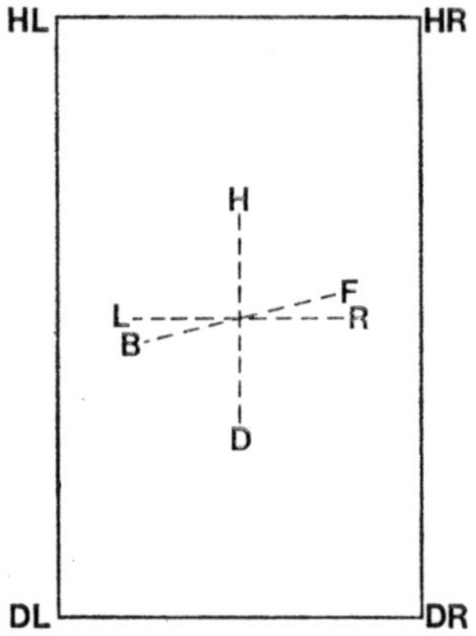

FIG. 13. The Door Plane

To continue:

opening while advancing leads to right forwards;
closing while retreating leads to left back;
opening while retreating leads to right back;
closing while advancing leads to left forwards.
The pathway linking these four points of orientation is known as the Table Plane (Fig. 14).

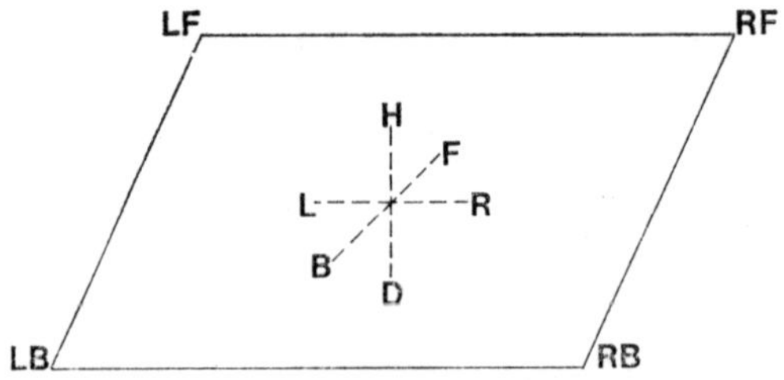

FIG. 14. The Table Plane

To continue:

advancing while sinking leads to deep forwards;
retreating while rising leads to high back;
retreating while sinking leads to deep back;
advancing while rising leads to high forwards.
The pathway linking these four points of orientation is known as the Wheel Plane (Fig. 15).

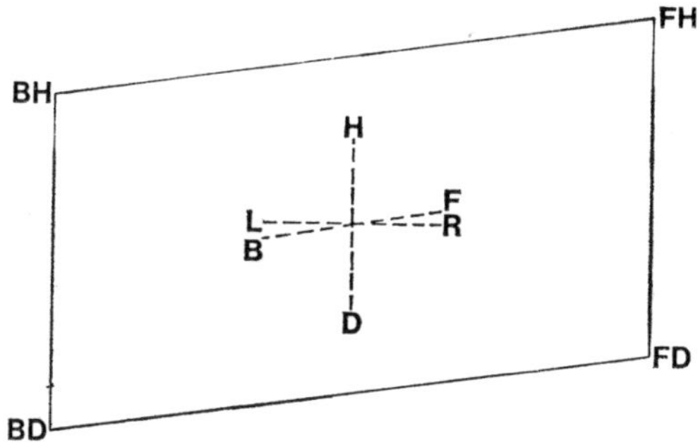

FIG. 15. The Wheel Plane

In all, twelve points of orientation have been arrived at in this way. If all these planes are linked to each other on the circumference we arrive at the shape of an icosahedron, shown in Fig. 16.

Many readers interested in movement will have come across models of this shape and wondered what it has to do with movement. If they consider the structure of the body they will realise its symmetry and how one side balances with the other, the upper part with the lower and the front with the back. Therefore, it is not surprising to discover that the natural body movements into the zones will, in fact, form this shape.

A sense of satisfaction is derived from moving in relation to these points of orientation in that one experiences the mobility of the diagonal stress without being too unbalanced and the stability of the dimensional stress without being too restricted.

It is useful to remember this section "pathways" as that part of the movement which answers the question, "Where into the space around me is the body moving?"

Rhythm

The variations of speed and placing of accents, the control of the flow of the movement and the flexibility and directness of movement, each alone and—as is most common—in combination, affect the rhythm of a movement and give it its particular quality and feeling. Everyone has a particular attitude to the

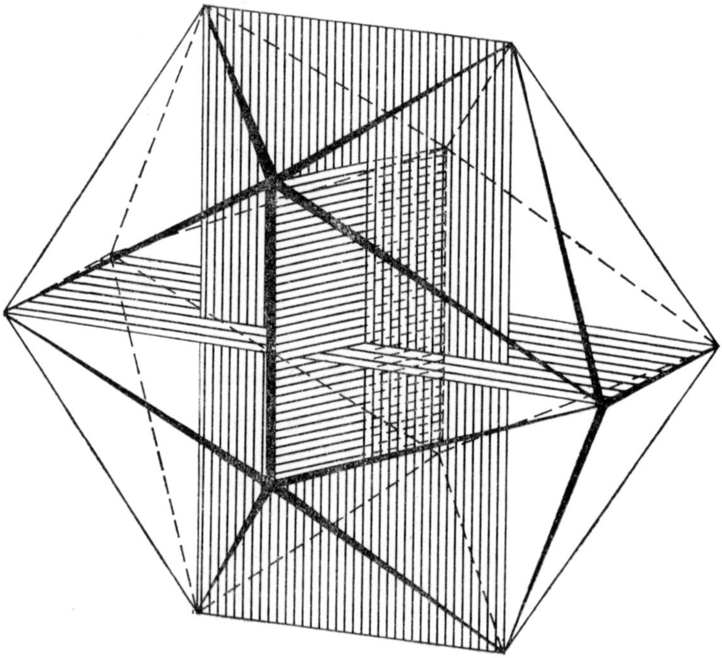

FIG. 16. The icosahedron, showing door, table and wheel planes

motion factors of weight, time, flow and space. Not only from the practical measurable point of view, but also indicating the inner participation and meaning of the movement quality. This could be a feeling of firmness and resolution, or sensitivity and gentleness. It could be a sense of urgency or shock as opposed to loitering or calmness. The person's attitude to space could be an economical one of getting directly to the point, or one of indulging in a meandering pathway. The movements may contain a feeling of holding back or proceeding with care as opposed to a bursting forth or a feeling of floating, care-free. These motion factors of weight, time, flow and space (in terms of quality) are described in more detail.

(*a*) *Weight.* Relaxation is brought about by complete absence of muscular tensions giving heaviness. Lightness or fine touch is obtained by overcoming the weight of the body and the pull of gravity in a delicate, buoyant, sensitive manner using appropriate muscular tension. Strength or firmness is obtained through resisting, fighting or utilising the body weight either against gravity or assisting it. These movements can be called strong, forceful, powerful, firm.

(*b*) *Time.* A movement performed in a minimum of time can be considered quick and described as sudden, urgent, sharp; one where performance is prolonged can be considered slow and described as sustained, legato, extended or lingering.

Variations of weight and time factors result in accents of movement. It is according to where, in a movement phrase, the accent is placed, that affects its rhythm and gives it its character. If placed at the beginning of a phrase it gives it an impulsive quality. An accent placed in the middle will give it a lift or momentum such as in swinging. A phrase where the accent comes at the end will build up to a climax, an impact, with a feeling of finality. In most movement phrases the accents arise naturally, but by being aware of them and emphasising them, a movement can be made very much more alive and interesting.

(*c*) *Flow.* The flow of movement may be continuous or broken and jerky. A movement that can be arrested at any moment can be considered bound and described as controlled, guided, restrained; one that can be stopped only with difficulty can be considered free and described as fluent, abandoned, unrestricted.

(*d*) *Space* (*effort*). A movement taking the shortest pathway from beginning to end can be considered direct and described as straight, undeviating, unwavering and economical in its use of space. One taking a winding pathway from beginning to end (three dimensional) can be considered flexible and described as twisting, meandering and indulgent in its use of space.

Combinations of the motion factors of weight, time and space form the basic effort actions as set out below.

Weight	*Time*	*Space*	*Action*
firm	sudden	direct	thrusting
firm	sudden	flexible	slashing
light	sustained	flexible	floating
light	sustained	direct	gliding
firm	sustained	flexible	wringing
firm	sustained	direct	pressing
light	sudden	flexible	flicking
light	sudden	direct	dabbing

There are two kinds of rhythm, metric and non-metric. Metric is measured and regular and is closely allied with stepping, such as in a movement of skipping and jumping:

Skip-Skip—Jump and turn
Skip-Skip—Jump and turn.

Non-metric rhythm is variable, it is the natural rhythm derived from gesturing, such as in a movement of gathering and scattering with variations in size:

Gathering in the right side of the body with the right hand and arm leading.
Scattering and turning with the left hand and arm leading with an impulse movement.
Gather both sides of the body while sinking.

It is useful to consider this section on "Rhythm" as that part of the movement which answers the question, "How is the body moving?"

COMBINATION OF PATHWAYS AND EFFORT. The teacher who has acquired an understanding of the basic elements of space and effort will readily be aware of the relationship between these and be able to make an apt choice of movement phrases to suit the level of the class.

The up/down dimension is concerned with changes of weight and effort. Muscular contraction in conjunction with the force of gravity makes for increased muscular tension. Release of muscle tension and expansion of the body, causing it to rise, produces light buoyant movements. Shock or surprise makes us spring backwards with suddenness, an instinctive protective action. The ability to see in front of us gives us confidence to move forward in a leisurely manner. The forwards and backwards dimension is concerned with changes of time. Extending sideways to the free side gives room for flexibility. Moving across to the opposite side brings restriction and makes the movement more direct. The side to side dimension is concerned with the direct and flexible qualities of movement.

The wise leader will make use of this information when introducing the basic elements of space and effort by devising movements which use them in their natural spacial areas. The eight corners of the cube formed by the diagonal cross help the teacher to cope with effort transitions and select movements based on the right blend of action, effort and space areas in order to obtain harmonious movement.

Relationships

All recreative movement classes should provide plenty of opportunity for mixing and working with others. Some of the most beneficial effects of recreative movement are experienced in this way. The activities (see the chapter on the body as an instrument) used by a group, influence the relationship as do the numbers involved.

(*a*) *Working alone.* The mover is concerned both with the relationship between one part of the body and another, such as the position of the elbow in relation to the opposite knee and with himself in relation to the space he is in. Even when working alone the mover is often in unison with the rest of the class and so situated as to enable awareness of the other members.

(*b*) *Working with a partner.* This is concerned with the relationship two people can have one with the other such as meeting, parting, passing, working together, following one another, mirroring and contrasting movements. Lifting and supporting would also be relevant here.

(*c*) *Working in threes.* Three people working together increases both the possibilities of formations such as circles, lines and triangles and also the variety of relationships in that they can move two against one, as well as in unison and in canon.

(*d*) *Working in a group.* These can be large or small and offer a variety of formations and relationship possibilities, *e.g.* a group of seven can move as a single unit or break up into three pairs and a one, or two threes and a one, a six and a one, or a five and a two.

(*e*) *Working in groups related to other groups.* This provides wonderful possibilities for interesting formations, working in unison, in contrast, in canon, merging, mixing, re-emerging and changing in numbers.

GROUP FORMATIONS. This is concerned with where in relationship to each other the group is placed and the formations this creates. Here it might be helpful to consider what some of these group formations are and the influence these have on the type of movement which emerges.

(*a*) *A cluster* of people (an irregular group shape) having no specific focal point, lends itself to development in various ways in response to the leader's task:

(1) in unison rising and sinking or swaying from side to side leading to travelling;

(2) the cluster can change its shape either by expanding and contracting or by following a leader in succession;

(3) a cluster can move with counter tensions within it;

(4) a cluster can weave and thread like a moving anthill (see Fig. 17).

(*b*) *Circle* (Fig. 18). Because the circle encloses an area it has an inward concentration making for immediate awareness for those making it and within it, but excluding everything outside it. In a circle there is no leader; all the members are

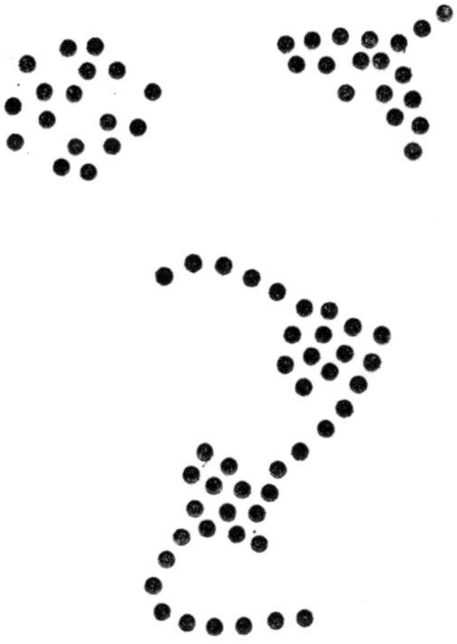

FIG. 17. The cluster

equal. Movements arising naturally from this formation are expanding and contracting, revolving, swinging, travelling and passing a movement on, *e.g.* a waterfall.

(*c*) *Line*—this can have many changing focal points which makes it extremely flexible. Used as a file, with one leading and others following can give rise to piercing, cutting movements, or a snake-like meandering about the space. It can at any time reverse the leadership so that the tail becomes the leader. It is

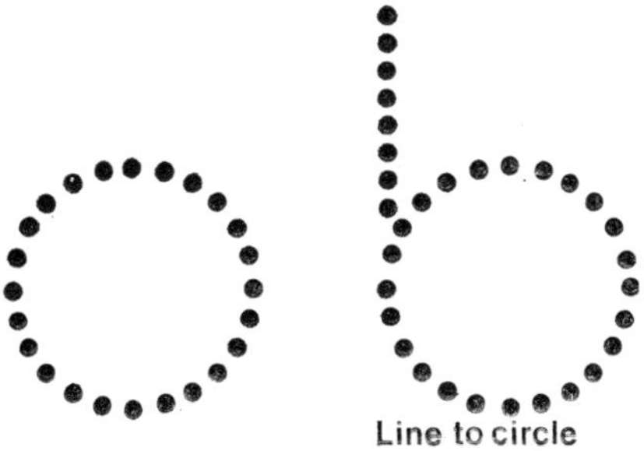

FIG. 18. The circle

easily changed into a rank giving a wall-like shape where the initiative is placed equally on each member. Movements arising would be rising and falling, advancing and retreating. The rank can expand or contract from one end, both ends or the centre. The line can divide and change itself into many shapes

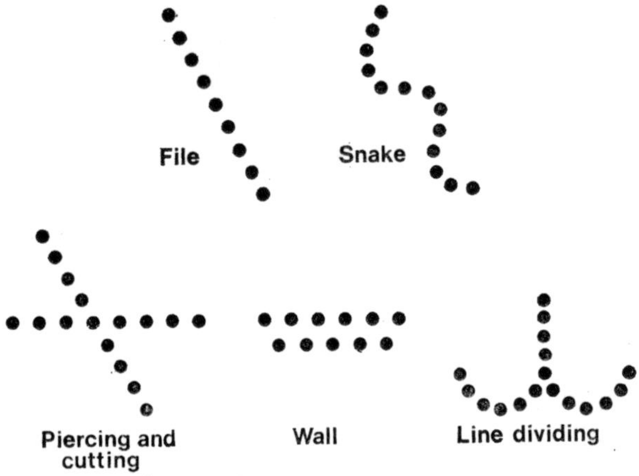

FIG. 19. The line

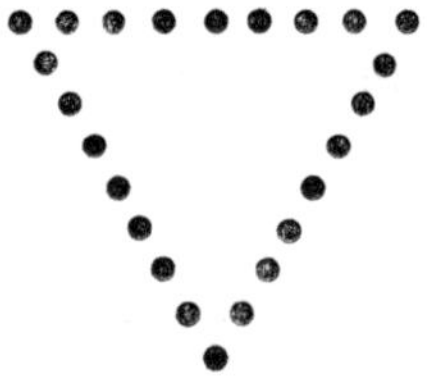

FIG. 20. The triangle

such as circle and crescent. The latter lends itself to enveloping without enclosing movements with an ebb and flow quality. Line formations are shown in Fig. 19.

(*d*) *Triangle* (Fig. 20)—this can be used as a spearhead implying direct, forceful, piercing action giving a sense of urgency. It also gives a choice of three focal points if the sides are considered, thus offering interesting changes of direction, especially when working in relation to other groups.

(*e*) *Square* (Fig. 21)—this is a powerful very symmetric, stable formation offering four focal points, each one containing a line of leaders who must work in unison. This restricts the choice of actions and produces mostly strong, formal ones.

FIG. 21. The square

It can be seen from the points made that certain group formations lend themselves more easily than others to inter-group relationships. The linear and cluster ones lend themselves to fast changing, flowing relationships while triangular groups relating to clusters or circles make for exciting, dynamic situations.

As well as the formations and numbers involved it should be remembered that the quality of movement chosen helps to determine different relationships. The qualities that we must consider are the group's attitude to weight, time, flow and space.

QUALITATIVE RELATIONSHIPS

(*a*) *Weight relationships*. Movements performed together with firm contact (mainly strong hand grips) give a powerful feeling of unity, creating confidence and a sense of belonging. It is therefore a good method of establishing group work with new members. Movements retaining a light touch are much more tentative, contact easily breaks and much greater sensitivity is required. This is, therefore, more difficult.

(*b*) *Time relationships*. The group has to learn to synchronise its movements to fit together without the help of accompaniment. In the early stages, actions involving stamping and/or clapping help members to hear the group timing. Later a group movement "playing with time" (slow and quick, sudden and sustained) or arriving together at one place, having started at different distances, demand a more difficult timing awareness.

(*c*) *Flow relationships*. This is the basis of communication and essential for recreative group activity. The flow of movement must pass freely from one to another as in an activity in which the members "pass on" a movement, *e.g.* a wave through a line or a circle. Catching, containing and passing on a simple movement phrase is a satisfying and pleasing activity. The use of small apparatus can be of help in the early stages of training this awareness.

(*d*) *Space relationships*. This is concerned with economy and extravagance in the use of space. A group moving with directness is purposeful, clear and economical. It is then that a feeling of unity is established and a decisive impact is made. Moving with flexibility creates diffusion. Transitory situations are difficult to maintain and require great sensitivity.

It is useful to consider this section "Relationships" as that part of the movement which answers the question, "Who are you working with?"

It cannot be stated often enough that it is not sufficient to read, talk or just observe movement in order to acquire a true understanding of what has been written so far. It is only through actually moving that one can gain a real knowledge of the kinesthetic, mental and inner personal experience that movement gives. With a real experience of the movement possibilities before us, we are able to remedy the limited and unbalanced movement range that the average person employs. We can strive for the mastery of movements of the body. We can increase its vocabulary and experience and widen the horizon of living. We can learn to observe to a greater depth to the benefit of others and ourselves. We have an unending combination of movement possibilities to explore and from which to compose movement sequences which can be physically beneficial and satisfying, stimulating to the mind and aesthetically pleasing.

Chapter Four

APPLICATION OF MOVEMENT

A BRIEF explanation of Laban's classification of movement as it applies to recreative movement has been given to help the teacher understand and meet the needs of the members. The first task is to be clear what these needs are. In this book we can only consider some generally applicable points but the teacher who gradually gains an intimate knowledge of the group will be able to relate these general points to the particular situation.

Motivation

On the whole it can be said that people join keep fit and recreative movement classes and stay with them for years for the following reasons:

(*a*) The satisfaction gained from physical exercise and the feeling that their bodies have worked, leading to an improved figure, increased muscle tone and a feeling of well-being.

(*b*) The need for relaxation by having a change of activity from their usual routine and a lessening of tension.

(*c*) To offset the boredom of a narrow confined way of living, *e.g.* bringing up a small family, lacking stimulation of reading and not meeting other adults, or a routine office job or other undemanding work. In other words the need for an outlet of pent-up mental and physical energy. For some it is the need to have an opportunity to invent and be creatively involved.

(*d*) To overcome loneliness, to meet different people and make new friends. To overcome shyness, diffidence, difficulty in communicating and to alleviate the need to gain more confidence. The need to contribute and participate in an activity which cannot be achieved alone.

(*e*) To satisfy the need for an aesthetic experience which is inherent in all of us.

There is no one activity which will supply the answer to one specific need. There is bound to be, and must be, an overlapping of effects in whatever activities are chosen. However, the following selection of activities show how some of the most obvious needs can be met.

APPLICATION ONE—PHYSICAL EFFECTS. "Ooh—ahh" this happy groaning is often heard following vigorous activity, especially when a teacher has been urging the class on to greater effort. But they would not be without this demand, for it is in this way their desire for and expectation of physical fitness is catered for. After a series of such lessons, members will be delighted to find that their breathlessness, aches and pains are vanishing.

What can we select from our movement content that will satisfy the physical needs of those who come to these classes? Obviously, the whole section concerned with "body awareness" and its activities (Chapter 3) will be of use, but it is the way it is used that will govern its effectiveness.

(*a*) Total extensions of the body will give an appreciation of a full stretch and complete contraction. This can be done from standing, lying, sitting, kneeling. The movements may be developed into travelling and jumping.

(*b*) The constant changes of body shape in twisting, elongating, curling and broadening, performed on different points of support, on the spot or in travelling, demand balance and control.

(*c*) Various ways of stepping and travelling with contrasting size and speeds on the feet and on different parts of the body give an appreciation of the management and strength required in locomotion.

(*d*) Combinations of the five basic jumps in a variety of rhythmic patterns make strenuous demands on the legs and call for stamina. Jumping is exciting and stimulating. Physical demands are increased if flight shapes are emphasised or landings are accented or held.

The above effects can be heightened in the following ways.

(*a*) The advantages of a repetitive swinging action are twofold, firstly it enables the flow of the movement to be felt, and secondly, it builds up a momentum of its own, which causes the body action to be extended beyond its previous range.

(*b*) Strengthening effects can be produced in an action, *e.g.* a whip turn or thrusting as in a kick. It can also be produced in stillness when arresting a movement, because the flow of movement has to be resisted. Asymmetric balances test muscle control and strength is required to maintain the static position.

(*c*) Jumping is one of the most strenuous activities in that it requires the sudden thrusting strength to lift the body into the air, balanced muscle tension to maintain the flight and muscular control to receive the weight in landing.

A common rhythm leading to work in unison influences the pace and continuity of the lesson, bringing a feeling of exhileration which stimulates further exertion. These activities need to be clearly directed by the teacher so that the class benefits from the security and feeling of unity.

APPLICATION TWO—THE NEED FOR RELAXATION. One of the reasons for the strain and physical tensions of modern life is that we no longer observe the rhythms of nature. In the past man rose with the sun, toiled while there was light and rested when dark. He worked according to the season of the year, whether hunting, tilling the soil, sowing or harvesting. If by the sea, he fished according to the ebb and flow of the tide, which in turn was governed by the rhythmic cycle of the moon.

His leisure was governed by days of worship and thanksgiving festivals of the season. There was time to pause and observe the results of his labour, to consider the task ahead and consider the miracle of the cycle of life—in fact re-creation. Twentieth century living has caused most of us to be largely independent of the harmonious pattern which was responsible for such a balanced way of life. Food is available at all times of the year, electricity lights our nights and replaces our primitive implements. The majority of us have been forced into areas of specialisation narrowing our outlook, interests and the physical demands made on us. In order to obtain relief and relaxation we should recognise the rhythmic balance of nature, the balance of contrasts—action and recovery, tension and release of tension, inhaling and exhaling.

With this basic knowledge the teacher must train the class through the process of movement in a way which will enable each person to achieve for themselves a state of mental and physical relaxation. Through the regular attendance at a recreative class they will be helped to appreciate the value that relaxation has for them and their families in daily living. Sound sleep will be induced if adequate preparation has been made through relaxation. Relaxed sleep allows the vital bodily repairs to proceed unhampered. Through the relaxation of muscular tension the body is able to minimise or rid itself of pain and even the fear of it. Irritability and despair can also be helped by physical relaxation and by acknowledging the need for change of occupation and thought, or even change of venue.

Pleasing conditions and warm, sympathetic teaching aid relaxation. To obtain this it is necessary for the body to be thoroughly warmed, to give the class members an appreciation of their body weight (heaviness) and the pull of gravity and the contrast of resistance to it. Movements which bring this about are:

(*a*) Systematic releasing of tension through one joint after another, separately or successively, from a standing position or floor-based. Taken to its full conclusion the body is completely relaxed—that is, inert.

(*b*) Following the natural rhythm of inhaling and exhaling which would lead the body into alternating tension and relaxation.

(*c*) Movements involving travelling or turning with swinging action will enhance the flow of the movement, promoting the release of tensions.

Clear, simple repetitive rhythms executed in unison in easy

formations such as a circle, give the movers confidence and time to adjust to the change from their daily situation. If this is taken in an informal, non-stop, follow-the-leader method of teaching this will assist the general mobilisation and achieve fully the objectives of limbering. Care must be taken that this section of the lesson is presented in a variety of ways in order to retain its freshness.

The theme chosen for each lesson will help to "flavour" the limbering (see lesson plan, Chapter 5). In this way the body is prepared for more demanding action and the mind made receptive. Relaxation or refreshment may be achieved by:

(*a*) being caught up in the pleasure of moving;
(*b*) meeting a variety of challenges;
(*c*) making a personal contribution;
(*d*) working with others.

If this very stimulating approach to relaxation of the body and mind is linked with the contrasts of body actions, efforts, spacial designs and groups, the change from one to the other produces a feeling of harmony which gives refreshment, especially when supported by appropriate music. For these effects to be properly beneficial it is important that a group remains reasonably constant over a period of time so that the members may gain from being together.

APPLICATION THREE—THE NEED TO OFF-SET BOREDOM. "I am so bored!" A typical indictment of living, and a sure sign that something is wrong. What are the symptoms of boredom? Weariness, heaviness, loneliness, apathy, indifference, lack of curiosity, lack of zest, lack of fulfilment. This a frightening picture, and yet we often hear it described. If we investigate the causes we find people caught by the monotony of routine, the sameness of surroundings or lack of objectives and initiative. Thus the vicious circle continues.

On the other hand, a person thrown into unfamiliar surroundings and a way of life where too many new demands are made can become so confused that the objectives become blurred, leaving a "rudderless" feeling, which also leads to boredom. Or it might even be a wealthy person surrounded by luxury, but because life lacks challenge he too can remain unfulfilled and again bored.

The concentration on body management centres interest on self, so increasing confidence. By becoming part of a group one is caught up in its enthusiasm, vitality and achievement, and gradually sensitivity to others will be awakened. Movements using travelling, turning and jumping with contrasting efforts of weight and time will give an invigorating and exhilarating experience. When playing with aspects of space such as levels, directions, air and floor patterns, space effort, direct and flexible movements, members of the class should become more aware of their surroundings and each other. The obvious way to cope with monotony is to ensure that there is variety in the work. This means variety within each activity, variety within methods of approach, variety in beginnings and endings of lessons. One way to achieve this is by making use of contrasts in movement, another is by doing something unexpected—creating a sense of surprise and a sense of fun.

Asking the class to achieve something almost impossible will help them to laugh at themselves. Giving them tasks involving agilities will challenge their sense of daring and doing something slightly daring is always exciting. Monotony can also be broken by the imaginative use of sound accompaniment. There are many ways in which a simple idea can be developed with variety, such as rising and sinking, for example with:

> different parts of the body leading, symmetry or asymmetry, jumping, opening and closing, travelling, turning, variations of time, variations of tensions, interruption, continuity, effort (direct or flexible), variations of size, changes of direction and pathways and relationship to others.

A mastery of any combination of these ways heightens and maintains interest while giving the satisfaction of achievement.

Another way of relieving boredom is to create situations in

which the class member can experience the excitement of discovery. The use of small apparatus is extremely helpful in this field, but the realisation of what the body alone can achieve is a revelation to many. Working with others introduces the class member to other peoples' effort rhythms. These may be very alien or contain ideas and opinions that are entirely new, thus widening their horizons and challenging their adaptability.

The talents of each member of the group contribute to the whole and the sense of purpose and belonging is increased if opportunity is given for these to be used outside the class situation. For example, some might like to organise a class outing. Others mount a display or arrange for a talk or demonstration to be given. The special interests of the class members can well be used to lead other members to be involved in the activities of the centre they attend or in outside events, and perhaps to increase their interests.

APPLICATION FOUR—GROUP WORK. The needs of the lonely, the shy and diffident, and those lacking in confidence and finding difficulty in communicating are largely met by those activities requiring two or more people and most of all when working in larger groups. There is no better way of getting to know others than by physically sharing, giving and adapting in a common movement.

It might be a group swirling, or rising and sinking, or circling, or even precipitating diagonally across the room. Immediately the individual is a part of the whole and belongs. The rhythm sweeps along and lifts the individuals out of themselves and their uncertainty—there is no time for self-consciousness, because their contribution is needed by others.

Over a period of time the effort of having to be a good group member brings increasing rewards. The sense of belonging grows into friendship, the need to contribute and finding the ability to do so gives confidence and the need to communicate in movement enables verbal approaches to be made more easily. For a group movement to be successful, every member has an individual role to play accurately, and this—though very rewarding—is also very demanding in a variety of ways, depending of course on the complexity of the group activity. Considerable expertise and ability to guide is needed by the teacher who might do well to create situations in which it is possible to clarify for the class what the different aspects of group participation demand. At the same time the teacher must be aware of and take account of those varied personalities and the needs they express either directly or indirectly.

For example, when clarifying the role of a leader in a simple task of following in travelling with changes of direction it may reveal the leader's inability to retain the followers. In this way the leader learns to make positive decisions concerning direction and rhythm and maintain them long enough for the group to "read" her intentions. The members of the file on the other hand have to be very awake and sensitive to what is happening and try to anticipate the leader's moves.

For a person to be "sensitive" she must call into play all her senses. She must observe, listen and feel. To do the latter she must have very light tension, "fine touch," particularly in her hands if this is how contact is established with others. For example, a loose group might be established in which all have very light contact one with the other and the task is rising and sinking. It will be through feeling her companions' movements that she will be able to adapt to the group rhythm.

For a contrast or even as an early group activity it is a good idea to have a group formation with a very firm contact, performing a clear, simple task—such as a circle formation with wrist grasp or elbows linking and a definite pattern such as circling left and right and coming in and out of the centre. This heightens the sense of belonging, the strong grip giving a feeling of support and security. The sense of hearing is heightened by group actions in which each member has to listen to and maintain the group rhythm, as for example in a loose group formation where the task is stamping or clapping with acceleration and deceleration.

Any group action which entails travelling, air patterns, coming together and parting, will necessitate close observation and if contact is made sensitivity through touch is immediately involved—for example, a loose group, all facing centre, contracting and expanding. When this is done playing with "time" as well—the group drawing together slowly and suddenly coming away—great demands are made on awareness if the group is to synchronise.

In order to enhance contact between people and help them to establish relationships, the flow of movement must be felt between them. It is as impossible to talk to a person who will not listen because she has "shut off" (bound flow) as it is impossible to understand a person who cannot "come out of herself" (bound flow.) It is through the flow of movement pouring inwards and outwards that communication is possible. So a wise leader will incorporate group activities in her programme where the flow factor is dominant—as for example passing on a movement, catching it and passing it on again, movements in which an action requires a re-action, a game of question and answer in movement.

As an introduction small apparatus could come into its own here—in actually passing a ball from one person to another, throwing it across the room or passing it along a line or circle. Alternatively, a crescent-shaped group without a ball could experience a wave-like movement passing through from one end to the other and then back again. Later, short movement phrases could be passed within a loose group formation.

Machine-like movements and movements derived from working actions where each person has a definite, if different, part to play within a complex whole and can identify this action with some outside objective can do much for those who suffer from self-consciousness. Working with a partner has many advantages. The member has only to lead or adapt to one other person. Each in turn has more opportunity to experience the responsibility of being a leader. Only one other person's wishes need to be considered and because of this creative activities are achieved more quickly.

The member has the opportunity of getting to know one person well and though perhaps she may be too shy to contribute in a large group, she may well contribute in a small unit, a particularly important point with regard to new members. It has its disadvantages, too, particularly for a new member. The partners might be incompatible, in which case the task may be too difficult and consequently both suffer from a sense of failure. Also one partner may be very confident and dominant, making the diffident one even more insecure. The over-dominant personality will benefit most in the larger group situation where the rhythm and pattern of movement will have a harmonising influence on the group relationship. The following situations can give opportunity for partner awareness.

(*a*) Follow the leader copying actions exactly.
(*b*) Watch the leader and do the opposite action.
(*c*) Work in unison with spontaneous reaction to one another.
(*d*) Trust the partner to lead whilst one's own eyes are closed.
(*e*) Reproduce rhythmic pattern made by the partner in sound or action.

The highest form of partner relationship is the evolvement of movements performed together where the leadership constantly changes. Here imperceptible communication through sensitivity must evolve so that each is able to anticipate and adapt to the other. Working with small apparatus in groups gives something tangible to work with and it is easier for the self-conscious to get absorbed and forget themselves. A great many requirements needed for group participation are most easily introduced by working with one other person in this way.

APPLICATION FIVE—AESTHETIC. Of the five basic needs referred to, the aesthetic is the most difficult to describe because it contains a quality least translatable into words. Phrases like "Man cannot live by bread alone," "Beauty is truth, truth beauty," may be an indication to some. Expressed in other words, it is man's need for enrichment by meaningful experience. Of course, what is meaningful and enriching for one may not necessarily be so for another and the media through which we find it vary tremendously.

An aesthetic experience may arise through creativity, the acquisition of skills, or a blending of both. Whatever form the experience takes it is one's ability to perceive, imagine and enjoy it as a whole, which makes it aesthetically satisfying. Recreative movement has much to offer in meeting this need for an aesthetic experience. It does so through feeling arising from movement, the visual enjoyment of shape and colour, the awareness of oneself as an integral part of a whole, recognition of the partnership of sound and movement and appreciation of textures.

The first of these—feelings arising from movement—can be illustrated by a sequence of movement involving rising and sinking with travelling and turning which gives satisfaction through the kinesthetic sense of mastery and flow of the whole phrase. In combining with a partner so that the two are working in opposition, *i.e.* A sinks to deep and B rises to high, the aesthetic satisfaction is increased by the feeling of sharing and the balance, giving harmony to the movement. This can be further enhanced by the class working in two groups. This same movement performed in two relating groups gives further satisfaction through being part of a meaningful whole. Although the majority of members are not consciously aware that part of the satisfaction in recreative movement is derived through this aesthetic experience, it nevertheless is the case.

The members are very quickly aware of their surroundings, whether they be aesthetically pleasing in proportions, lighting, colouring, texture and, most important of all, cleanliness, or the reverse. Over a period of time they may become increasingly aware of the existence and value of surroundings in their more abstract forms.

We are aware of the inherent need to create in every one of us and with a thoughtful approach to teaching, situations can frequently be provided to enable those who wish to avail themselves of the opportunity to create. This may well be one of the main contributions recreative movement will have to make in the future to retain the interest and satisfaction of its members.

Chapter Five

THE LESSON

WHEN the lesson is no longer based on the anatomical structure of the body, but on the development of a movement idea, a different attitude and method have to be applied. This does not imply that the anatomical structure of the body is not considered or that care is not taken that all parts are equally exercised, through movements in which all parts work naturally and harmoniously as a whole.

Planning

Having decided on the theme according to the ability of the class, Fig. 22 shows the curve of progression in a lesson. How it starts gradually, builds up to a climax and is brought down to a quiet, calming finish. The increase of demand is not only in physical expenditure, but also mental concentration and

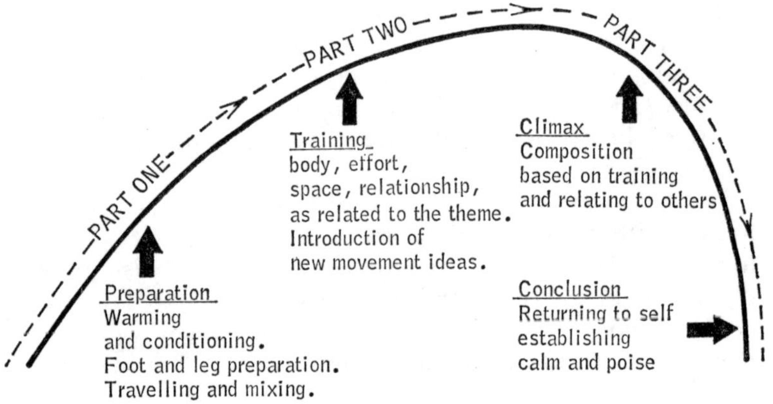

FIG. 22. A lesson curve

absorption at the same time as having to adapt and work with other people.

(*a*) *Part one—Preparatory activities.* Before doing any strenuous physical activity it is vital that the body should be thoroughly warm and "oiled" as it were—properly prepared for any strain or stress which it might be called upon to undertake. Warmth will go a long way to provide this as it will relax the body. Bodily warmth will be created by any activity which promotes the circulation such as friction, rubbing, slapping, clapping and easy bending and stretching activities which cause the muscles to act like a pump on the veins and push the blood back to the heart. Swinging and circling movements will mobilise the joints and relax any tension which would inhibit movement.

It is necessary to have movements which strengthen as well; stretching followed by a collapse (yawning and release) is a good preparatory activity and any pulling, pushing and strong holding actions will promote strength in the muscles. Relaxation (release of tension) is essential, in between, to allow for recovery. Particular care must be taken to give the feet and the legs adequate preparation, as they do have to work very hard throughout the session. These preparatory activities should lead to some travelling sequences involving simple space awareness, and particularly awareness of the other class members.

Throughout this section the teacher should not only be concerned with the physical preparedness of the members but ensure that the social side is catered for, by placing the class in such a manner that they are able to see each other as well as the teacher, such as a circle or semi-circle with the teacher in the centre. Opportunity must be provided for moving off the spot, seeing and meeting other people and seeing a different aspect of the room. In other words, a chance to get the feel of the whole situation. The introductory session should be carefully worked out to be worthwhile without being too demanding physically or mentally. The movements should be simple to achieve, short in duration, require little coaching and not too much concentration. The final travelling and mixing activity should have a simple completion in itself, creating a small climax within the lesson and establishing a light, happy atmosphere.

(*b*) *Part two—training*. The next stage builds on to this good foundation by getting to the heart of the matter. Its essence is the training of body awareness to improve bodily skill in order to promote quality and variety within movement phrases. There should be a series of these, each one becoming more demanding, and all giving the experience required for the main climax of the lesson. It is at this stage that the teacher's acute observation is very necessary so that the class can be coached on the main aspects of the theme. Ideally this theme should be approached in all sorts of different ways so that members not only achieve the satisfaction of mastering the task but also understanding the quality and feel of the basic movement idea. Attention, concentration and pertinacity should be demanded from the class. Repetition is good as long as it is still purposeful and the class is not too tired. Within this section, too, will be moments of climaxes and recovery. Short breaks may be incorporated, giving a release of tension and concentration, so preventing too much intensity.

(*c*) *Part three—climax*. So, gradually, the lesson progresses to its climax. This should be the peak of the session, fully implementing and challenging the experience gained. It should provide an opportunity for working with others to create a composition. The satisfaction gained at this stage of the lesson should come from the personal mastery of the sequence, playing one's part within the group interpretation and so participating in the final achievement.

Having enjoyed this experience the class member needs to return to self. Generally speaking, the aim should be for a calming-down effect, leaving the member with a poise indicating his or her physical and mental well-being. In certain instances, if the climax has had a particularly quiet and slow quality, it might be necessary for the final activity to have a livening and releasing effect as an antidote to deep concentration.

TIMING. New leaders may be concerned with the proportion of

time given to each phase of the plan. It is suggested that in a session of approximately an hour the timing could be roughly:

ten to fifteen minutes for part one;
twenty to twenty-five minutes for part two;
twenty to twenty-five minutes for part three;
three to five minutes for conclusion.

The order in which a lesson is prepared is immaterial and would vary for many reasons. Sometimes it is useful to start with part one and develop the theme towards the climax. At another, it will be more stimulating to start by planning the climax and selecting the work that builds up to it. At other times the teacher may wish to emphasise the training aspect of movement, in which case part two will be considered first, so that the limbering will be the preparation for the training aspect and the climax will be its implementation.

When thinking in terms of a purely creative situation it might be advisable to have a freer approach, so that ideas can develop spontaneously from the interaction between the teacher and the class. The emphasis in this type of work is on the composition and its expressive quality.

THINKING ROUND A THEME

The first task, therefore, is to consider the needs of the member and what aspects of movement will fulfil these needs. This gives the basic movement idea or theme. For example:

(*a*) In a new class where the important thing is to get to know each other and feel relaxed in each other's company, the theme would be all those activities and situations which would promote opportunities for meeting, mixing and ensuring an awareness of the whole group. "Meeting and parting and passing through", "over and under and round about", would be suitable movement themes.

(*b*) Members of a class who are tentative and lack confidence need to experience what they can do with their bodies and to trust themselves to do it. They need to experience the feeling of committing their weight to the floor and exploring the space around them; in other words, emphasis on body awareness in weight transference and carrying the body in different areas around them. A suitable theme to cover this need would be "weight transference and levels", "rising, sinking with rolling and turning." Study of the movement section, together with good class observation, will suggest further movement ideas.

A theme is a movement idea around which the lesson is built, increasing its sense of purpose and guiding its development. It is suggested that the teacher has available a large sheet of paper on which to jot down any ideas immediately they occur. As can be seen in Fig. 23 a whole hotchpotch of ideas has become intermingled with the basic classifications given in this book and it can be seen how one idea triggers off another, overlaps and connects. Some teachers might find it helpful to use one or more subsidiary themes. This could help in guiding selection and ensure a good balance within it. Another way of ensuring that all aspects of movement have been taken into consideration is to check whether there is something on that sheet of paper which answers the questions, "What?" "Where?" "How?" and "With whom?"

The next task is to make a suitable selection according to:

(*a*) the type of class;
(*b*) the experience of the class;
(*c*) the conditions of the working space;
(*d*) the length of the lesson;
(*e*) the temperature of the room.

Thinking aloud in this way enables the teacher to become fully involved in the movement possibilities of the theme, so acquiring confidence when teaching, to draw upon material for coaching purposes which might not have been selected for use when the final preparation was completed.

Such complete preparation allows for a change in mid-stream should something prove to be unsuccessful. So it is from

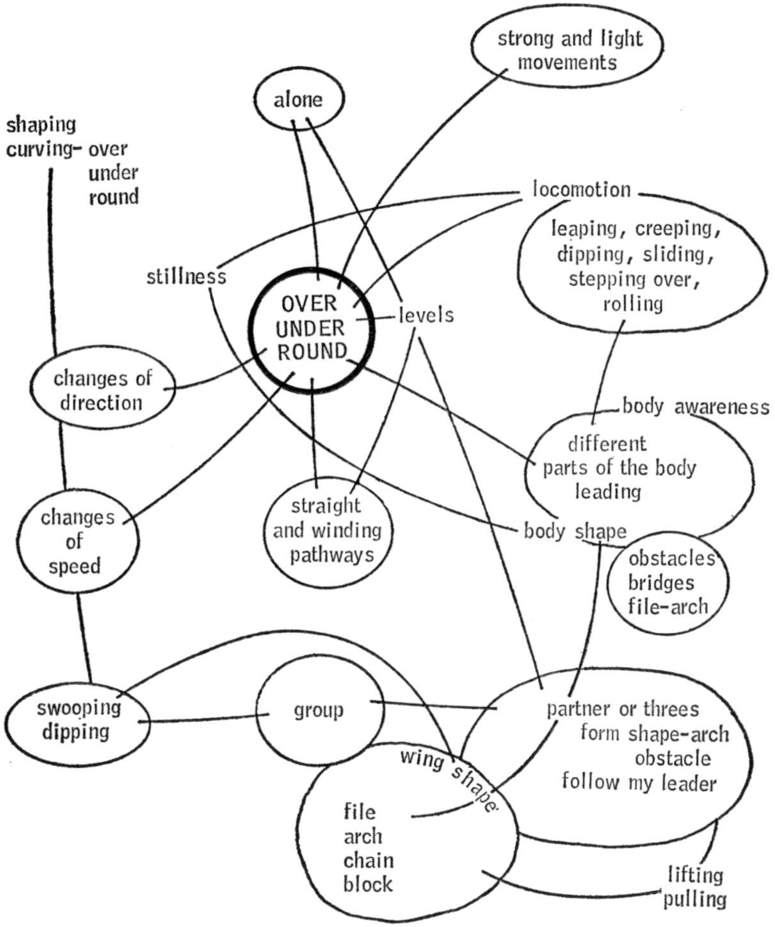

FIG. 23. "Hotch-potch" of ideas to aid selection

this rough sketch that suitable work for each section of the lesson curve has to be selected, but always with reserves and variations in store. Here are thirteen examples of themes that can be considered. Examined carefully, it will be seen that there are many aspects inherent in each, the richness of which can be extended according to personal choice in the way shown in Fig. 23.

high, low and turning;
pushing, pulling and scattering;
swaying, circling and spreading;
the feet, the hands and top of the head;
above, below and encircling;
leaping, subsiding and meandering;
alone, together, moving and still;
increase, decrease of body activity, size, time or effort;
twining and piercing;
separating and gathering;
jagged and smooth;
enlarging and diminishing;
economical and extravagant;

PLANNING CHECK. Having planned the lesson beforehand, presenting it should be considered in the light of its proportions and continuity. It will be helpful for the teacher to consider this under the following headings:

(*a*) *Physical*—does the lesson give opportunity for use of the whole body on the spot and in travelling?

(*b*) *Rhythm*—is there variety in rhythm and phrasing?

(*c*) *Space*—are there variety of levels, changes of direction, size and variation of patterns?

(*d*) *Social*—are there adequate opportunities to work alone and with others?

CONTENT OF A SERIES OF LESSONS. In deciding the content of a series of lessons the teacher has the choice of working on a substantial theme for a number of lessons, or a slighter one for a single lesson. The word slighter does not imply that it is of less value. If working on a more substantial theme it is not enough that the lesson should just be repeated: certain aspects within it should be changed to add variety and extend the experience. At the same time a good deal of the material should be retained to give the opportunity for improvement of performance by repetition.

In moving on to a new theme the teacher is able to link it

with previous experience by recalling movements from it and using them in a new setting. A check should be kept on the balance of new and familiar work so that the class is neither bored nor confused, but has a feeling of progression. Should the teacher feel that the class is not responding to the theme, it would be wise to change it.

ASSESSMENT OF A SINGLE LESSON. Having taken the class the teacher should assess the results to decide how far the class has responded to the teaching and to what degree the aims of the lesson were achieved. The following questions might help:

(*a*) Did the class enjoy the session?

(*b*) Did they find the work challenging and satisfying and did they finish with a feeling of exhilaration?

(*c*) Has their bodily skill been improved and has their resilience and poise increased?

(*d*) Has their adaptability to the space and their sensitivity to others improved as the class progressed?

(*e*) Did the variety of rhythms, class arrangements and the opportunity for social contact help to make the class successful? Did all the members have an opportunity to make a contribution?

(*f*) Did the music heighten the general enjoyment of the session?

If the answer to any of the above is no, the teacher should try to pin-point the cause. This could be:

(1) unsuitable choice of work;
(2) inadequate presentation;
(3) inadequate and poor accompaniment;
(4) circumstances outside the teacher's control.

Having discovered the cause, the teacher should be able to plan accordingly for the next lesson.

Progression

To discover whether the class is making satisfactory progress the teacher must be able to stand back every now and again to assess the work. This is done by watching, by checking the content of the lessons and by considering what happened in the light of what should have been achieved.

Certain factors should be evident after a few weeks. There should be an improvement in the relationship between the teacher and the class and between the individual members, leading to greater confidence and trust. The members should have developed a sense of personal responsibility to the group and be prepared to use their own initiative to deal with small needs such as opening windows, tidying up, or making tea. The members should be able to respond quickly to the teacher, work with some sensitivity to each other, and make the best use of the space available.

DEVELOPMENT OF THEMES. To retain interest and a sense of satisfaction class members must be aware of the constant challenge to achieve greater mastery of their bodies. This they can do by extending their physical range as well as by improving their understanding of the movement vocabulary. It is essential for this movement vocabulary to be presented in a logical order. It would be unwise to choose a theme dealing with effort actions when the class has not mastered combinations of simple body activities. In the initial stages the themes chosen should concentrate on:

(*a*) Body management—transference of weight;
symmetrical and asymmetrical movements;
body shapes;
body flow;
combinations of body activities.

When concerned with handling small apparatus and other materials it is essential that the function of these is recognised and mastered before creating movement phrases:

(*b*) aspects of space— space words;
away, towards, around, near, far;
levels;

air and floor patterns;
directions.

(*c*) elementary rhythms—simple combinations of strong and light tensions;
quick and slow speeds;
continuous and broken movements.

(*d*) easy relationships— awareness of others in the room;
keeping a common rhythm;
working with or against a partner;
working as a group on any simple aspect just mentioned.

Group participation demands concentration and therefore it is essential that to begin with, the task given is limited to one aspect at a time. The group must be allowed to establish itself before the movement content is made more complicated.

When the level of work has been firmly established the class may be introduced to more complex themes. A teacher who has studied the class members' needs will be able to select suitable themes to cater for these, as in Chapter 6.

The needs will be complex and the order in which the teacher elects to deal with them will itself form a progression.

PROGRESSION OF MOVEMENT ACTIVITIES. Let us now consider how the movements themselves are introduced. An easy movement phrase is one which is short, concerned with one movement idea, performed on the spot and in the easiest balance situation. It can be introduced either as a whole body movement or through the medium of the hands, before putting the stress on other body parts. Body parts should be moving in their own spatial zones. A fairly slow and regular rhythm is easy to follow.

Taking these points it is easy to see how any simple idea may be developed and made more challenging. Of course, one or two changes will be quite challenging enough and it would be unwise to increase the difficulties too quickly. Ways of developing a movement are as follows:

(*a*) The movement phrase could be lengthened.

(*b*) There could be a combination of movement ideas.

(*c*) The movement could be made to travel.

(*d*) The balance could be made more difficult.

(*e*) Two or more body parts might be stressed or made to move simultaneously.

(*f*) Body parts might be made to move out of their natural spatial zones, *e.g.* the legs leading the movement into the air and the arms making a gathering gesture near the floor.

(*g*) The movements may be performed more quickly, the rhythms made more unusual and irregular.

(*h*) From being easy, the movements could be made more physically demanding.

Other ways which increase the challenge of the work are to demand a greater movement memory by stressing exact repetition of movement phrases and longer sequences, or to demand greater clarity of what every part of the body is doing and how and where it is moving in space.

So far consideration has only been given to progression of movement by an individual working alone. As soon as another person is involved a number of other factors have to be taken into consideration. The merits and demerits of working with a partner or a group of people have been gone into in detail in Chapter Three.

Figure 24 gives an example of a lesson plan. It will be noted that the comments column is empty—its purpose is to enable the teacher to record an immediate assessment of what has occurred, which should then give guidance for procedure in the following lesson. This could form the basis of a single lesson or a number of lessons. There are several ways in which this can be done:

(*a*) The lesson may be repeated as it stands in order to concentrate on those coaching points not covered the first time. In addition, the standard expected of the class could be raised.

(*b*) The climax could be developed in a variety of ways:

(1) change from unison to working in canon.

(2) keep the pattern intact, but give emphasis to a specific aspect, such as effort quality.

(3) keep the same pattern, but work as a group relating to another group.

(*c*) One of the movement phrases enjoyed in part 2 could be developed as the climax for the ensuing week, thus giving a different emphasis to the lesson.

(*d*) Keep the movement content the same, but change the accompaniment to some or all parts of the lesson.

Keeping a file

Every teacher will find it invaluable to keep a record of the work undertaken by each class. A working file will clarify the teacher's thinking, assisting consideration of what has been done, planning what is to be attempted and assessing progress made. The record should include facts and information about the classes with an indication of their requirements; plans for each week's work, with assessments of achievements and failures and any other points that may have arisen from time to time in thinking about the development of the group. It will also form a record of work for those responsible for organising the class. Recording is a means of clarifying aims and thinking and so enables one to teach with confidence and skill.

In the working file the teacher can keep items of information which will help with the organisation of work, such as:

(*a*) Names and addresses of organisations from which information, books or equipment may be obtained.

(*b*) Particulars of equipment such as the weights, sizes or types of small apparatus, balls, hoops, music records and other materials.

(*c*) Details of reference books—where they can be obtained and their main points of value.

(*d*) Notes, original or cyclostyled from training courses which would be valuable for quick reference.

This file should serve as a starting point when the teacher is

FIG. 24. An example lesson showing the tabulation method of recording

THEME — OVER — UNDER — ROUND

Lesson Plan	*Movement Content*	*Purpose*	*Coaching*	*Accompaniment*	*Comments*
PREPARATION Conditioning	Shaking body parts, high and low	Increase circulation	Vigorous with feeling for body weight	Strong beat, lively perhaps familiar	
Mobilising	Swing high, drop low Swing into circling arms, legs	Increase suppleness of the large muscles maintaining full range of joints	Use of body weight to achieve impetus and full size of movement	Three rhythm pendulum then impulse accents	
Strengthening	Stretching as in a yawn, sustained closing	Improve muscle tone	Maintain pressure and resistance in the muscle joints	Two rhythm with firm steady quality	
Foot and leg work	Ankle joint bend, stretch, circling, stepping high and deep	Strengthening ankle, knee and hip joints	Full range of movement at the ankle. Sensitivity of the feet	Two rhythm, jaunty. Two rhythm, strong and light touch	
Travelling and Intermingling	Travelling high and low around or over others	Familiarise with space and awareness of others	Awareness of rise and fall pathway and recognition of people	Flowing three rhythm	

Lesson Plan	*Movement Content*	*Purpose*	*Coaching*	*Accompaniment*	*Comments*
TRAINING Body Training including Quality of Movement and Spatial Considerations	Lift over, scoop under, scatter round	Mastery of the body in rising and falling. Flow of the movement achievement of design	Awareness of levity and gravity. Continuity and air pattern. Extension into open turn at medium level	Change of melody	
	Step over, roll under, travel around	Mastery of the body elevation and transference of weight leading to agility	Lift of leg action transition of on to the floor and off the floor. Awareness of focal point	Two rhythm underlining the power and staccato quality	
	Jump over, thread through, follow the leader roundabout	Mastery of jumping. Learning to work with others. Awareness of shapes and spaces	Coaching take-off flight and landing. Awareness of body parts leading and body shapes. Sensitivity to leadership. Choice of pathway	Three rhythm. Three phrased pattern, strong staccato accent on first phrase and diminishing effort in following too	
CLIMAX	Group in unison facing the same way. Travelling (going over and under), rising and falling, spreading and closing while turning	Experience of working in group. Opportunity of using experience gained during lesson	Awareness of relationship within the group. Clarity of floor and air pattern	Repeat of flowing three rhythm on pattern of three phrases	
Conclusion	Repetition of lift over, scoop under, scatter round, individually	Return the individual to themselves. Establish feeling of gaiety.		Light mazurka.	

looking for stimulation and inspiration. Personal notes made on movement or about practical sessions which gave great pleasure can give a boost to thought when re-read and through this mental limbering the mind is prepared for further planning. It is useful to collect lists of movement words, which, when rolled off the tongue, provide a fresh angle on something familiar. Thirty different words meaning "quick" or "slow" are bound to suggest colour in movement. Visual things will spark a chain of fresh ideas; magazine photographs whose grouping, quality or attitude catch the eye will give a new way of considering a movement.

Stimulation need not necessarily be derived from a movement basis. Sometimes we come across points so aptly and vividly expressed that it helps to collect them as quotes so that they can be kept before the mind. Ways of working and attitudes are often expressed by people we meet, live or on television, or in a play. These are just examples of how the mind can be stimulated. Every person will be interested by different things that, for them, would be worth noting.

A file, to be useful to its owner, needs to be a personal thing and tailor-made to fit the special situations in which the teacher works. Allowing one's own way of thinking and working to come through reflects a personal attitude at that time.

The file will grow as experiences multiply. It needs to have order and clarity, but not necessarily uniformity and clinical tidiness. It should not be a collection of other people's cyclostyled notes, though these have their place in the reference section. The size and style of the file is a matter of the teacher's individual choice, but it needs to be easy to handle, have a contents list or reference guide and simple form of classification. Colour can give it life and appeal but what is most important of all is that a file is a symbol of the teacher's achievement and therefore something to take pride in keeping well.

Presentation

Presentation involves the changing of the lesson plan from words on paper into a comprehensive sequence of movement phrases which ensure a build-up from the simple and familiar to the more challenging physical and mental demands of the climax. Although the lesson has three phases (see Fig. 22), the teacher must present it with continuity, giving it a sense of wholeness, within which a series of climaxes may arise, adding contrast of pace and rhythm. The form of the presentation will be influenced by the movement to be taught and the needs and ability of the class members.

Many factors affect the individual's ability to learn. Temperament is an important one; those with a tendency to anxiety, or who are withdrawn, will find movement more difficult to achieve than the out-going extrovert. Experience in other fields of learning will help people to be more receptive, those used to changes in their lives will probably be more adaptable and flexible to new methods of teaching. Some will be quick to learn, others slow; some are easily discouraged, others like to be strongly challenged.

For these reasons the teacher needs a many-sided approach in introducing the work to the class. An imaginative vocabulary with variety of inflexion and modulation in the voice will help. Constant sensitivity to the class members and their reactions are also necessary to make the lesson successful.

The following methods are ways of introducing the work to a class. It is the skilful interplay of these methods that adds to the enjoyment by retaining the interest.

IMITATION. The teacher demonstrates and the class copies. This may be follow-the-leader style where the teacher works with the class as in limbering, or it may be a demonstration by the teacher or a selected person or persons, which the class observes and then copies. The advantage of this method is that the class has an immediate picture of what is required and so is quick into action. It creates a oneness between the teacher and class, giving a feeling of security. The danger lies in a badly performed demonstration or poor observation, causing the class to acquire bad habits of moving. Demonstration dictates that everyone will be moving in unison, so this method is unsuitable if the teacher wishes the class to make their own contribution.

INSTRUCTION. The teacher leads the class by carefully chosen words through each stage of the movement phrase, thus making them think it out for themselves. This allows for individual interpretation within the task set and leaves the teacher free to observe and the member to concentrate on the mastery of the movement. It is necessary to be brief, using action words and allowing the tone of the voice to indicate the quality of the action.

The variety of response increases the necessity for skilful observation. The teacher must make sure the class is fulfilling the task and performing to a high standard. If it is not, the teacher must observe why and give the necessary coaching.

REPETITION. This may be the use of familiar work to get the class going and to give a feeling of security, warmth and gaiety, or the practice necessary to master new movement situations or achieve aesthetic satisfaction from the polished performance of a movement study. Repetition here serves a useful purpose, but used indiscriminately it produces boredom and a decline in performance.

EXPLORATION AND DISCOVERY. In this situation the class members are given the opportunity to discover for themselves the possibilities of a task. With judicious choice of task this is a method that any teacher with any class can use at some point. It throws the member on his or her own resources, giving an opportunity for contributions, stimulating initiative and—if working in groups—promoting leadership. It makes great demands on the teacher's judgement. The task chosen must be within the ability and understanding of the members, otherwise they will feel inadequate. They must be given freedom to work, but be helped to achieve their ideas. The great variety of work will test the teacher's powers of observation and skill to coach helpfully without limiting each individual's effort. The teacher should try to keep a freshness of approach by making use of different stimuli.

For example a movement can be initiated by rhythm pattern. A clap or step determines the rhythm which is then developed into travelling and turning. Another time the movement can start from the study of the space design and the development be concerned with the qualities within that design. A club will give a fresh approach to swinging movements which will easily develop into travelling, turning and jumping. A scarf will help movers feel the qualities of floating, sinking and whipping. The sharpness of a clave sound underlines a staccato movement, while the ring of a cymbal can help sustainment.

Movement can be described, demonstrated, experienced and observed. Using several of the senses helps to reinforce the learning. When introducing a movement to the class it is wise to start from something that is simple and familiar and then develop it, bringing in the new aspect with plenty of repetition. If care is taken to introduce only one new difficulty at a time, the class can master this thoroughly before moving on to the next and the lesson does not become over-loaded leaving the students with a feeling of inadequacy. If there is a feeling of planned, logical development to the lesson, students will feel happy and more confident in the teacher and in their own ability. When there is a demand for strong concentration at some point, it is important to follow it with a lighter approach towards something easier to achieve, thus making a contrast and ensuring the best response from the class members.

There is a danger in reaching the objective too quickly and thereby losing the quality of the whole. It is unwise to teach a complex study or sequence without breaking it down and analysing its various components, so that each can be clarified and mastered. This can be done as a preparation for the presentation of the whole. However, if for the sake of achieving the mood or expression, it is taught in its entirety, analysis and practice should follow, before repeating it again. It cannot be stated often enough that whatever method the teacher chooses to present the work, it is the quality of the relationship between the teacher and the class that makes for success or failure.

Observation and clarification

One of the skills of teaching is the ability to react to what is seen. In order to see fully, the teacher must be free of personal anxieties and moods. Experience of observing people is needed and it is possible to train oneself in this by constant practice, observing people in general situations outside the class perhaps at work or when travelling on public transport. It cannot be emphasised too strongly that it does require conscious practice and, of course, knowledge and experience of the subject matter is essential to good observation. Most of the time during group work, the teacher needs to stand back in order to evaluate each group's achievement.

To make observation purposeful it helps to look at one particular aspect at a time.

(*a*) people—individually and as a group
(*b*) facilities and conditions
(*c*) the movement

(*a*) *People.* Observe the physical condition of the class members. Are any of them overweight, elderly, in robust health, cold or out-of-health? If any of these conditions are observed it is necessary for the teacher to take them into account when planning her work and react to them. For example, if the class members are cold, use movements aimed at stimulating circulation. Overweight members' attention could be drawn to the literature available on slimming and general health.

Notice the mood of the class—are they withdrawn, reserved, boisterous, bubbly and over-excited, tired, depressed or aggressive? A positive and optimistic attitude will help here. The teacher should set this atmosphere in the class and perhaps link the movements to working either in home, factory, office or shop so that the members are helped to maintain this attitude during the week. Class members who arrive tired or harassed should be given time to put aside the demands of home or work and adjust to concentrating on themselves as people responding to class teaching. They should be soothed by feeling the support of the teacher's care during the mobilisation section. The pace of the lesson may be more leisurely, giving time for coaching and achievement, or the teacher may decide to lift the class out of their tiredness by the sparkle of the lesson. Here care would be taken in the choice of movements to see that they were predominantly ones which were accented upwards with lightness, and with the opening actions preferably in simple situations using gay rhythms. Movements which accent space, design and relationship will help to refresh tired members.

Lastly it is important to observe the way the members relate to one another. Are they isolated, in cliques or happily integrated? For selecting situations which will encourage interrelationships, see Chapter Three.

(*b*) *Facilities*. Observe the conditions for working and the space available. Are the floor surfaces safe and the walls free from protruding objects? Are the movements suitable to the space available and the floor conditions? (See also Chapter One.) Overcrowding or an awkward-shaped room would mean that the teacher must give special care to the placing and class arrangements, both for the safety and the satisfaction of the class members. For example, travelling movements with emphasis on distance or speed would be frustrating in a crowded room, but a feeling of space can be created by arranging for the class to travel down the room or for half to work at a time. Travelling and turning movements with a feeling for space could be adapted by emphasising rhythm rather than space.

(*c*) *Observation of movement*. As has previously been said, the teacher's first job is to observe whether the class has understood the task given. If not, it is necessary either to repeat the instructions, or better still to find another way of presenting them. Assuming that the instructions have been understood, the teacher should then be ready to observe the degrees of mastery of the movement. A new teacher may find it helpful to compare the best and weakest movers to assist observation and decide on coaching action.

It will help the teacher to make observation purposeful if the habit is formed of looking for one specific aspect at a time and these would most sensibly come under the following headings:

(*a*) body,
(*b*) pathways,

(*c*) rhythm,
(*d*) relationship.

Each of these aspects may be observed generally over the whole class or in individuals. Under each heading we have suggested the kind of questions it would be helpful to ask and then looked at ways of finding the answers.

OBSERVATION OF THE BODY. What is the starting position? Is the movement one-sided or two-sided? What part is receiving the weight? What is leading? Which part is stressed? Do the feet assist the movement? Is the knee bent or stretched?

There are several ways for the teacher to set about clarifying these points. If a common movement pattern is being directed the task is to ensure that each member conforms. This can be done by repeating the instructions, demonstrating or questioning. Certainly in an informal situation where members have selected their own movement, pertinent questioning will be necessary to make them clarify what they are doing. Another method is to ask two people to match their movement phrase or to observe one another.

For more subtle observations such as the reasons behind the lack of elevation in a jump, one would question what preparation has been made for the jump or whether there are any dead areas in the flow of movement through the body. The teacher can use movement training to draw attention to that part of the body which has not been participating and then practise its performance. The teacher must draw on movement understanding to diagnose difficulties—this involves being able to see the separate parts of the whole.

OBSERVATION OF PATHWAYS. Where is the movement taking you—forwards or backwards, high, medium, deep, inward or outward? Can you draw the air pattern and/or the floor pattern? The teacher helps in this clarification by checking positions in space and so developing a kinesthetic sense, directing observation and helping to define the shape, by moving slowly and with greater control.

OBSERVATION OF RHYTHM. How did you travel to your partner—swiftly or reluctantly? Was there an accent? If so, where was it placed? Can you clap the rhythm of the movement? Here the teacher's task is to help decisions to be made about intentions by:

(*a*) clarifying the instructions;
(*b*) helping the understanding of the quality through examples and practice;
(*c*) listening to the rhythm or music;
(*d*) discussing the quality and repeating the movement.

OBSERVATION OF RELATIONSHIPS. With whom are you working? When are you alone and when are you related? What is the quality of the relationship—strong and binding or tentative? In this aspect the teacher needs to foster the required feeling by using very simple activities in easy situations which awaken sensitivity to others. Not until this feeling is established is it wise to increase the numbers of the group or the complexity of the movement. Should the group activity fail it will be necessary to simplify it in order to correct the fault. An apt vocabulary will help to stimulate the mood required.

So far we have been considering observation and coaching under specific headings, but in the teaching situation, the problem is to see the movement phrase or study as a whole. It is from this that an analysis of the difficulties has to be made and the priorities for coaching decided. The following example may help to show how this can be done.

The movement is run, jump, turn and land. Difficulties could be in take-off, flight and landing.

(*a*) Training movements could be given on basic springs, body shapes in the air and receiving weight, all practised separately. Then a return would be made to the original movement phrase.

(*b*) If observation showed that mastery was still inadequate, the teacher could simplify the phrase by taking out the turn and leaving the jump.

(*c*) If observation showed that the phrase was easily achieved, she could increase the challenge. For example, run into jump, jump, jump, roll and stand.

No teacher can hope to rectify all the faults of poor performance in one lesson. It must be recognised that the majority of the basic skills in body management can only be improved over a long period of regular training. Experience will help to achieve the right balance of coaching to ensure enjoyment and satisfaction. It is important to be selective and sensitive to the class reactions when making corrections. Coaching is only successful if it it is constructive and inspires the members to improve.

Chapter Six

STIMULI

CONSCIOUSLY or unconsciously, movement imagination is stimulated by the impressions received through our senses of the ever-changing world. Visually we are affected by shape, colour and texture in nature, architecture and the pictorial arts. Aurally we are bombarded by music, words and sounds that may be concordant or discordant. Physical contact with the elements of nature and in the handling of many shapes and textures, natural and man-made, enriches our awareness of the environment. Conscious use of these impressions may enrich movement vocabulary, which, when employed in creative work, will in its turn develop a deeper understanding and sensitivity to our surroundings.

The following notes suggest some ways in which movement may be studied through the aural, tactile and visual senses.

Aural

An early satisfaction for man was the exuberance and exhilaration gained from feeling his own body rhythms. Through the experiencing and repetition of these natural rhythms he became aware of the sounds his own body produced such as clapping and stamping. Often the feeling evoked by the movement caused him to shout, shriek and hiss. These discoveries led him to the conscious use of song, words and percussive sound and the realisation that he could use these to evoke emotional response in others as well as himself.

Therefore, in studying sound and rhythm it will be useful to start by using rhythmical body sounds. Movers should be encouraged to clap, stamp, click, brush, scrape, hum, whistle, grunt, whisper and murmur as an accompaniment to their own improvised movement. Percussion instruments can be used to pick up any of these rhythms or to act as a stimulus for new ones. The tambour, clave, cymbal and bells all have their own sound quality which inspire corresponding qualities in movement. The varied rhythmic patterns that can be made with percussion instruments have a compelling, vital effect upon the movement which gives great pleasure to the performers. The following tabulation shows the division of familiar percussion instruments according to the sounds they produce and the corresponding quality of movement.

DRUMMING SOUNDS	*Movement qualities*
drums tambours bongos	very versatile, textures vary according to the way the instrument is played, have strong rhythmic quality.
SHARP HARD SOUNDS	
wood blocks claves temple blocks clappers castanets scrapers	jerky, angular, direct, restricted, thrust, flick, dab
RINGING SOUNDS	
Indian cymbals bells triangles chime bars tubular bells gongs large cymbals	going on, suspension, impulse and fade, strong to delicate, tendency to curving
SHAKING SOUNDS	
maraccas chocolas tambourines sleigh bells	vibrating, pulsating

MELODIC SOUNDS	
chime bars	
swanee whistles	strong suggestion of spatial awareness,
glockenspiels	
xylophones	according to the instrument and the
plucked strings	way it is played, all qualities can be achieved

The teacher and the class members will find it exciting to discover the variety of sounds they can produce on any of these instruments according to the way they are handled and the kind of beaters used. They will find that some instruments are restricting and others more versatile. A greater variety of stimuli can be obtained by grouping or orchestrating the sounds. This field can be widened still further by introducing musical compositions.

USES OF AURAL STIMULI. Music and movement are so closely linked that they complement one another and it is possible to interchange their roles of leading and following as desired. In order to follow and complement the movement, a musician with the ability to improvise and compose is essential. In this way the rhythm pattern and space design of the movement composition is enhanced, without losing any of its character.

It is important in any new movement experience that the rhythm of the action be thoroughly felt before introducing accompaniment. Similarly, in evolving a movement composition it is essential for the movers to experience and establish the rhythmic pattern which arises naturally from this particular composition. This may be so satisfying that accompaniment is unnecessary. If it is decided to use some form of accompaniment, care must be taken to ensure that it follows the rhythm, shape and quality of the study exactly.

When the movers are working to a musical composition, care must be taken to study its rhythm, phrasing and form, style and melodic line. The movers must transform the composition into their own medium, as they understand it. The kind of music chosen is dependent upon the taste of the individual. The teacher must be sure not only to satisfy personal taste, but also to be aware of the musical preferences of members and the suitability of selections to the kind of movement to be done. Variety is therefore essential in two ways:

(*a*) in shape, rhythm and qualities which stimulate movement ideas and support the theme of the lesson;
(*b*) in the style of the music, *e.g.* popular, classical or light.

If selecting a passage from a large composition it is important to ensure that the section chosen is complete in its own right. When combining passages from different compositions care must be taken in the selection both from the point of the musical form and the movement composition. It is advisable to select the passages from the same composition or at least from pieces by the same composer.

The success of the music and movement partnership will depend upon the quality of the relationship between the teacher, pianist and the movers. As with any other relationship this requires sensitivity to one another, respect for one another's discipline and contribution, and the ability to be adaptable. This team work needs establishing in small practical ways and must be given time to mature. The pianist is an integral part of the class.

The most versatile instrument of all is the human voice. To make full use of this requires some tuition and practice. The tonal quality of the voice affects the movement response in the same way as a musical instrument does. It sets the mood and atmosphere of the class and care must be taken that it does not have the adverse effect of being irritating or inaudible.

Words should be chosen with care for their power to stimulate immediate movement response. A rich vocabulary will encourage creativity in movement. Groups of action words can be the stimulus for a movement phrase or movement study. For example:

flying, hovering, bursting;
tossing, curling, collapsing;

drifting, darting;
swinging, flying, circling.

The rhythm and shape of a poem as well as its mood and content can provide inspiration for an individual or group study. Songs can also be used in this way.

THE USE OF TAPE-RECORDINGS. It must be clearly understood that a tape recorder cannot replace live accompaniment, but as a means of providing a change or making it possible to have orchestral music, it is a great asset. In a case of emergency when the pianist is absent its value cannot be over-estimated. It is important, however, that it is used judiciously and that the recordings are good. The advantage of a tape recorder is that music can be "caught" at any time from different media. A catchy melody from radio or television or a friend's record may be used, or a private session with a pianist improvising for a movement study may be recorded. It may sometimes be useful to record music from a performance for future reference or practice. Teachers are however advised to acquaint themselves with the restrictions of copyright concerning tape recordings.

Taping music from records prevents their wear and tear and allows for easy repetition of the exact phrase. It is also possible to select passages from long-playing records. When teaching with a tape recorder it is useful to break the music up into phrases, in the same way as a movement composition is broken up. These music phrases could easily be recorded many times so that repetition of the movement is possible without having to re-wind the tape. Having music on a tape enables the teachers to prepare and practise for their sessions at any time.

There is no easier way of carrying a large selection of music than on a tape, but it is vital that a careful index of the material on the tape is kept under the following headings:

index number; title; composer; orchestration; use.

Such a record helps the teacher to find the particular piece of music required quickly and should the tape be damaged, the source can be easily found and a new recording made. No doubt over a period of time, the teacher will find that music has been used for other purposes than the original one. It is advisable to make a note of all the different uses made of each piece. For example:

The Aquarium—Carnival of Animals—St.-Saëns
(*a*) sustained and continuous;
(*b*) travelling and on the spot;
(*c*) travelling and turning, with rising and sinking;
(*d*) individuals, partners and groups

In order to be equipped with a wide repertoire of music for movement, it is essential for the teacher to listen to as much as possible, as often as possible and to all types of music that are available such as classical, light orchestral, popular, folk, electronic and film. In order to use this repertoire well the teacher must learn to select wisely and with discrimination to give the class the widest possible movement experience.

Tactile

One of the ways man comes to terms with his environment is through the instinctive need to touch and feel and so understand and be able to communicate with the world around him. This can be seen in the normal behaviour of people, especially children. The prevalence of "do not touch" notices in museums, exhibitions and shops is evidence of this innate desire in us all. Some modern art sets out to satisfy this craving by encouraging tactile and physical exploration. Handling such varied objects, natural and man-made, as feathers, stones, gauze, wood, ribbon, balls, hoops and rope, calls for differing body actions. The quality of the movement is influenced by size, shape, rigidity or pliability and the texture which might be slippery, spiky, convoluted or flat. The following notes may help with the planning of practical work.

BALLS can be: bounced
thrown
caught

rolled
balanced

They can be manipulated by: one hand
two hands
the feet

Using the ball to perform these actions helps the mover to:

(*a*) develop resilience;
(*b*) stretch, curl and twist, making various body shapes;
(*c*) be aware of the relationship in space between the ball and the body, *i.e.* away, towards, around the body or parts of the body;
(*d*) develop skill in handling and contacting the ball with different body parts and to have the opportunity for movement involving one side or both sides of the body;
(*e*) use transference of weight, steps, locomotion, jumps, turns and stillness.

Each of the above actions can be thought of in conjunction with:

(*a*) the way in which the body is involved, *i.e.* throwing with the feet, catching with the hands;
(*b*) the use being made of the space, *e.g.* bounced low, bounced high, or thrown side to side passing overhead;
(*c*) how the ball is handled, *i.e.* how fast or slowly it can be bounced, how softly or strongly it can be thrown or caught. How it can be used with claps or bounces in order to make rhythmic patterns;
(*d*) handling the ball alone or with others, *e.g.* rolling the ball along the floor to a partner, picking it up and throwing high before repeating the movement. Each person can have a ball so they are exchanged or one ball can be used;
(*e*) performing a movement phrase with the ball either in unison or in canon with a partner, in a trio or a quartet.

Ball work should lead to lively, dynamic, quick moving, fluent movement.

HOOPS can be: rotated (edge or surface leading)
thrown and caught
spun
rolled
climbed through

Hoops may be manipulated by:

(*a*) one hand but the free flowing movement obtained makes the hoops more difficult to control;
(*b*) two hands which restricts the movement of the arms and so leads to greater spinal movement.

Using the hoop to perform these actions helps the mover to:

(*a*) stretch, curl and twist, making various body shapes calling for spinal mobility and strength;
(*b*) use transference of weight, steps, locomotion, jumps, turns and stillness;
(*c*) develop skill in manipulating the hoop and become aware of its position in relation to the body.

Each of the above actions can be thought of in conjunction with:

(*a*) the body action which is required, *e.g.* spinning the hoop, changing from right to left hand and back without checking the hoop spin, or swinging the hoop to take the mover into travelling and turning;
(*b*) where the hoop is used in space, *e.g.* thrown, caught and spun away, towards and around the body;
(*c*) how is the hoop handled, *e.g.* with changing speeds when spinning the hoop and with a stronger pull. When circling the hoop overhead a quick light change of grip is needed;
(*d*) with whom are you working, *e.g.* partners can be joined together by two hoops. They can rotate, turn, tilt and move the hoop so that movers are led into travelling and turning. Groups of four can be linked together by a hoop,

swaying and rotating in the circle using their weight to pull the circle into different shapes.

Hoops lead to excellent spatial movements.

CLUBS can be: swung
thrown and caught
balanced
guided
rolled
used to make percussive sounds

They may be manipulated by one or two hands holding either the narrow or bulbous end. Using the club to perform the above actions helps the mover to:

(*a*) accomplish transference of weight, take steps, jumps, turns and be still;
(*b*) be resilient;
(*c*) bend, stretch and twist, so making varied body shapes;
(*d*) develop skill in manipulating the club and be aware of its position in relation to the body and space around it.

Each of the above actions can be thought of in conjunction with:

(*a*) the way the body is involved, *e.g.* increasing the swing of the club to give impetus to a circle turn, perhaps with a jump;
(*b*) what use can be made of space, *e.g.* swinging the club high to the ceiling, letting it fall directly to the floor, the hand and the body dropping with it;
(*c*) how the club is handled. It can be held lightly in the finger tips or strongly gripped, *e.g.* an easy preparatory swing away and back leading into a strong slashing action and ending with a light tap on the floor;
(*d*) working with others, even though with a club this is difficult. It can most simply be done by using the club to

make percussive sounds, *e.g.* holding the bulbous end and making rhythmic patterns against the shaft of the partner's club forcing a backwards or turning movement. One rhythm pattern could be made with the partner's club and one on the floor travelling to meet a new partner.

Work with clubs leads to dynamic movements.

MATERIAL of different weights, textures and colours used in different shapes and sizes will give opportunity for very varied movement responses. It can be made to:

(*a*) float, undulate, flutter;
(*b*) whip or flick;
(*c*) slide, drag or slither;
(*d*) take tension and support weight.

Because material is soft and pliable it can be handled in a great variety of ways, with one hand or two. Making material do the things listed leads the mover to:

(*a*) change body shape;
(*b*) transfer weight, travel, turn, jump and be still;
(*c*) be aware of the shapes that can be made with the material and how they relate to the body and the space;
(*d*) be sensitive in re-acting to the effort and speeds required to move the material.

Each of the above actions can be thought of in conjunction with:

(*a*) the way the body is involved *e.g.* two or three people holding the edge of the material resting on the floor, all close to the floor. They rise sharply to send the material billowing in the air and sink to the floor at the same speed as the material;
(*b*) the use which is made of the space *e.g.* three people holding the edge of material firmly with one hand pulling outwards to make the material taut. Working in canon and

keeping the tension, they move under, round or over others to change the shape and vary the level of the material;

(*c*) how the material is handled. This can be any way from a finger tip touch to a strong grip that is taken with suddenness or sustainment, smoothly or jerkily, *e.g.* holding the material by one hand so that it trails, moving to keep it air-borne, experimenting to see how slowly, quickly, strongly or delicately it can be moved or its pathway changed.

According to the size and weight of the material it can be manipulated by an individual, partners or a group. Because of its easy handling the movers are free to relate to one another through the material in diverse and original ways. Handling material suggests and encourages an excellent variety of movement qualities, even with beginners. The possibilities of work with materials are endless. They add another dimension to movement in providing variety, exhilaration and enjoyment.

It is hoped that the manipulative skill acquired through the handling of all these objects will carry over into everyday handling. Certainly there is no doubt about the sense of achievement arrived at by this kind of mastery. Consideration needs to be given to the placing and timing of such work within a general scheme. It helps beginners to avoid self-consciousness by directing their attention to an outside object. If the objects are carefully chosen they will give experience in various qualities of movement. It gives an immediate sense of achievement if the handling is successful. With the more experienced mover, working in this media helps to give refreshment by a change of emphasis. For those who have considerable mastery of movement and depth of knowledge, this work gives added challenge and discipline.

Visual

The impact of a visual stimulus tells so much so quickly and so succinctly. One sees the mood, the form and the relatedness of the whole in a flash. It evokes an immediate response which quickens the imagination. The swirling and eddying of water, the tossing and quivering of leaves and branches, the leap of a flame, the flash of a fish suggest movement actions that have rhythm. Pictures, sculptures, rock formations and other natural objects suggest shape and form for individual and group movements. Colour and lighting convey mood and can influence the quality of a movement.

It is obvious from these word pictures that the study of the various visual stimuli leads naturally to expressive work. The chosen object needs to be scrutinised sensitively in order to discern its essence. Discussion will reveal the diversity of reaction to what is seen, and if working in a group, a decision has to be taken on the basic ideas to be explored. A period of undirected study will be required to find what aspects of the movement vocabulary will express the meaning of the initial inspiration. It is from these that a selection of one, two or three simple movement statements is made. By repetition and varied development within a clear form the composition acquires a life of its own. Such compositions may arise from any external stimuli, as well as from movement motifs.

Conclusion

Here we are brought to the threshold of creative dance composition, an art form in its own right, which might well add another dimension to recreative movement. This is not to belittle the values of movement for physical fitness and exercise, on the contrary it is important that the emphasis should be on a variety of approaches if recreative movement's value to a wide public is not to be restricted.

Much of this book has been concerned with the practicalities of applying the principles, which indicates the value we place on them. The fact that this last chapter on stimuli draws attention to the possibility of the work having potential as an art form is an expression of belief on our part. We hope others may at least consider and perhaps accept this belief. Whether that is so or not we hope to have given enough guidance to make this the practical handbook it is intended to be.

Appendix I

DEMONSTRATIONS

Open classes.

The dictionary definition of a rally is a participation, a banding together to make common cause, a rapid re-union for concentrated effort. A rally serves to create a feeling of belonging and of unity, to achieve good standards of dress, movement and behaviour and to establish friendship links between individuals from different parts of the country. It could have detrimental effects too. A rally takes the form of a recreative lesson, but because of the very large numbers, strong accent on the social occasion and the fact that the teacher has a restricted time to function with this expectant group and surrounding audience, means that there is a danger that the quality of the work done will be sacrificed to playing to the gallery. The teachers and members may also be misled into thinking that this is how a weekly class should be taken, instead of realising that this is a special presentation for a special occasion.

An open class brings together people with very different movement vocabularies, so the lesson needs to be planned in such a way that everyone can have a sense of achievement. Movement phrases which give a choice of performance will please both the beginner and the experienced mover.

There are many new unfamiliar factors for the movers to cope with in such a class, so the movement, rhythm and the music accompaniment could be the unifying influence if they are chosen with care. Whatever the theme of the lesson, some participants will have come primarily to meet others, so there must be ample opportunities for them to do this in easy movement situations that they can master and enjoy. Open classes usually have some form of audience so the teacher needs to consider the visual look of the lesson. This is most easily achieved by considering the group arrangements. The most effective ones are usually the simplest and with careful planning beforehand the teacher can make good use of these very easily. It is as well to remember that some movements which are good to do in the privacy of a class are not ideal to watch. Clothing must be thought of in terms of its visual impact too.

Open classes can only be successful social gatherings when great care has been put into the planning stages and the following details taken care of:

(*a*) There should be clear travel directions to the building being used, adequate car parking facilities, and an entrance for welcoming and checking members as they arrive.

(*b*) Changing facilities should be roomy and warm with places for clothes, good washing facilities and lavatories.

(*c*) The hall should be broad as well as long, with a raised area from which the teacher can be easily seen. A microphone—a collar one if possible—should be provided if the numbers are very large or the acoustics poor. The floor should be smooth, clean and not slippery and the ceiling high and with adequate overhead space.

(*d*) The programme should be carefully thought out and publicised with good clear announcements throughout. It should be so planned that the final part works to a climax of togetherness and is not allowed to tail off leaving the members and teacher with a feeling of inadequacy and disappointment.

(*e*) If guests are invited, those responsible should see that they are comfortably seated with a good view, but not in such a way as to intrude on the movers. They should be publicly welcomed and whenever possible introduced as individuals as this helps to give a feeling of unity and understanding.

(*f*) If serving refreshments, however simple, adequate spacing with plenty of servers will avoid delay and frustration. Seating should be considered and litter can be avoided by good planning.

(*g*) As with an ordinary class first-aid facilities should be available and the nearest telephone noted.

A well-planned, happily executed programme should send

everyone home with a wonderful feeling of stimulation and achievement.

Demonstrations

Demonstrations can be classified according to the audience, the place and the purpose of the occasion. This may be informal or formal. Usually the purpose of informal demonstrations is to publicise the work in order to win support for the activity or to provide an audience for a group who need this stimulus to bring their work to fruition. The formal demonstration is used to entertain and to act as a shop window for the type of work presented, giving amateur groups the opportunity to work towards a professional standard.

(*a*) *Informal movement demonstrations.* The main aim here is to establish a warm relationship with each member of the audience in order to persuade them that recreative movement is something each one could do, enjoy and benefit from. The audience needs to feel at one with the members demonstrating, so it is best to work in the round. By talking to the audience as well as the class, the teacher helps to unite them into a group. This is further achieved by choosing simple activities which those in the audience would feel were within their capacity to perform. It is important that demonstrators should be suitably dressed and well groomed and aware of their general bearing and poise.

They should be well briefed about the purpose of the demonstration so that they are able to speak with confidence to members of the audience. It is good for members of this type of demonstration to be a cross section of a typical recreative class so that members can identify with someone demonstrating. A short talk about the movement often precedes this type of demonstration which should include short varied items. Even though it is an informal demonstration, it is important that it should be well organised and of a high standard.

(*b*) *Formal movement demonstrations.* These can be divided into three main categories and though the main aim of each is entertainment, the standard of work is very much to the fore and is of great importance. The categories are:

(1) small demonstrations with the accent on excellent performers and sound movement content;

(2) large demonstrations to be performed in large halls before a big audience with the accent here on spectacle, design, colour and mobility;

(3) outdoor demonstrations which are also dependent on colour, patterns and mobility with unity and directness to project their effect against the "great out-doors."

In planning any of these kinds of demonstrations the following factors have to be considered:

(*a*) The physical shape and size of the area to be worked in—it is important to have the exact measurements so that the work can be planned to make use of the shape available;

(*b*) The position of the spectators and their relation to the working area and whether they are placed above, below or level with the performers. The movement must be planned so that the audience has the most effective view;

(*c*) Texture and colouring of the floor, which is particularly important if the audience is looking down. Planning the colour of the costumes is relevant here and also the colour of any props or apparatus to be used. This is particularly important when working on grass;

(*d*) The number of entrances and exits available and what is the most effective use of them to underline the character and quality of the item presented. Outdoor demonstrations require a single wide entrance in order to make an impact;

(*e*) Timing of the parts and the whole. Single items need to be short, leaving the audience wanting more. These items need to be varied and contrasting. Each one will have impact if it is planned on a theme or idea with a starting point, a development leading to a climax or through a series of climaxes to the main climax and the resolution;

(*f*) The visual effect on the audience. The performers need to be carefully selected for their movement ability and their suitability for the role they are to play. The number taking part needs to be carefully considered having regard to the size of the demonstrating area and the groupings required. The fewer the performers the greater need for good movement and appearance. When larger groups are presented the movement ability of each individual is not so conspicuous. Larger numbers provide opportunity for greater varieties of pattern or grouping. This is more effective in larger areas and out of doors, particularly when seen from above. Colour of costumes can also help in enhancing pattern changes, especially if courage and imagination contribute to the choice and underline the mood and impact of the item;

(*g*) Lighting, if it is used, must complement the movement by creating atmosphere or high-lighting movement climaxes. It should not obscure the movers or endeavour to cover their inadequacies. The primary function of any lighting effect is to light up the movers;

(*h*) Sound—it is essential that the quality of the sound is good and audible, also that the amplification speakers are well placed. This is particularly important out-of-doors where there is competition fron extraneous noises.

Care chould be taken that the choice of accompaniment relates to the mood of the movement composition, the actions involved and the number of performers.

Demonstrations can be fun to do. They make great demands on the enthusiasm and tenacity of the participants and can raise the standard of performance. They should be used to stimulate the general work of the class, but not allowed to dominate it.

Appendix II

Addresses of organisations, societies and governing bodies

Central Council for Health Education, Tavistock House North, Tavistock Square, London WC1

Imperial Society of Teachers of Dancing Incorporated, 70 Gloucester Place, London W1

Keep Fit Association. *General Secretary*—Mrs. J. Worrall, 26 Park Crescent, London W1N 3PB

Information concerning training courses and Leader's Award

Laban Art of Movement Guild. *Hon. Secretary*—Miss E. A. Osgathorp, 6, Regency Court, Sittingbourne, Kent

The Physical Education Association of Great Britain and Northern Ireland, Ling House, 10 Nottingham Place, London W1M 4AX

Sports Council, 26 Park Crescent, London W1N 3PB

British Red Cross Society, 9 Grosvenor Crescent, London SW1

Books for Further Reference

ABERCROMBIE, M. L. J.: *The Anatomy of Judgment* (Pelican)

COOKE, DERYCK: *Language of Music* (Oxford Paperbacks)

COPLAND, AARON: *What to Listen for in Music* (Mentor Books; Pub. New American Library)

EKLUNDH, MARGIT: *Spare your Back* (Duckworth & Co. Ltd.)

HUBBARD, D. V.: *Your Body and how it Works, No. 1* (Edward Arnold Ltd.)

MATHEWS, WENDY, *and* WELLS, DILYS: *Nutrition* (Home Economics and Domestic Science Review, London)

NEWSON, OLIVE: *Skipping* (Keep Fit Association)

ROGERS, JENNIFER: *Adults Learning* (Penguin)

SMITH BRINDLE, REGINALD: *Contemporary Percussion* (Oxford University Press)

ULLMANN, LISA (Editor): *Rudolf Laban speaks about Movement and Dance* (Laban Art of Movement Centre)

WARD GARDENER: *New advanced First Aid*

Bibliography

ANDERSON, MCLURG: *Housework with Ease* (The Scottish Council of Physical Recreation)

LABAN, R. *and* LAWRENCE, F. C.: *Effort* (Macdonald & Evans Ltd.)

LABAN, R.: *Modern Educational Dance* (Macdonald & Evans Ltd.)

NORTH, MARION: *An Introduction to Movement Study and Teaching* (Macdonald & Evans Ltd.)

PRESTON-DUNLOP, VALERIE: *Handbook for Modern Educational Dance* (Macdonald & Evans Ltd.)

ROGERS, J. (Editor): *Teaching on Equal Terms* (B.B.C. Publications)

RUSSELL, JOAN: *Creative Dance in the Primary School* (Macdonald & Evans Ltd.)

KEEP FIT ASSOCIATION: *Scheme of Training*

H.M.S.O.: *Principles of Anatomy and Physiology for P.T. Instructors*

INDEX

Accents, 33
Achievements, 2, 4, 6
Advancing and retreating, 28
Aesthetic, 40, 50, 51
Air patterns, 27
Anatomy, 6
Assessment, 59, 63
Asymmetry, 25, 43
Aural stimuli, 75, 77

Balance/off balance, 8, 18, 28–29, 31, 42, 44, 51
Ball and socket joint, 13
Ball work, 80, 81
Body, structure and function, 6–21
  alignment, 17–18
  instrument, 23
  activities, 23–25
  awareness, 25, 54
  shape, 4, 26
  flow, 26

Circulation, 11, 16, 19, 53
Clarification of movement, 25, 63, 69
Climax, 53–54
Clothing, 3
Clubs, 83, 84
Communication, 23, 47, 49
Companionship, xiii, xiv, 2, 47
Confidence, 45–46, 47, 48, 49, 50, 55, 56
Contraction, 15, 16, 35, 42
Cumulative strain, 18, 20

Demonstrations, 87–91
Development, 42, 43, 46, 60–63
Diagonal cross, 28
Digestive system, 18
Dimensional cross, 27
Direct movement, 33, 35, 40
Directions, 27
Discovery, 47

Effort, 34, 42
Elevation, 24
Equipment, 2–3
Evaluation, 59, 60
Exercise, 19, 41, 42
Extension, 42, 43

Facilities, 2, 71, 88
Feet, 4, 10, 11, 17, 53
File, 63
First aid, 21
Fitness, xiv, 42
Flexible movement, 33, 35, 40
Flow, 26, 33, 40, 43–44, 49, 51

Gesture, 23, 25, 34
Gliding joints, 14
Groups, 36, 39, 47, 48, 61

Hands, 10, 11, 25
Harmony, 43, 45, 50, 51
Heat regulation, 19
Hinge joint, 13
Hoops, 82, 83

Icosahedron, 31, 32

Joints, description, 11, 12
  types, 13
  movement of, 26
Jumping, 24, 43

Keep Fit, xiii

Laban, vi, xiv, 22
Lesson, 52, 62–65
Levels, 27
Lifting and carrying, 20
Limbering, 16, 45, 53
Locomotion, 24, 42

Materials, 84, 85
Membership, 1–3, 55, 56
Metabolic rate, 18
Mobility, 31
Mobilisation, 11, 45, 53
Motivation, 1, 2, 41
Movement phrases, 26, 42–44, 61–62
  examples, 34, 65
Muscles, description, 14–16
  function, 15
  tone, 16, 17, 18
Music, 77–78

Nutrition, 17, 18

Observation, 22, 48, 59–60, 68, 59–74
Octahedron, 28
Open class, 87
Opening and closing, 38

Partnerwork, 35, 49–50
Pathways, 26, 35
Pelvic girdle, 9
Percussion, 76
Peripheral movement, 28, 29, 30, 31
Planes, 29, 31
Planning, 52, 58
Posture, 17, 19
Preparation, 4, 55, 57
Presentation, 3, 66–69, 87–89
Progression, 52, 58, 60, 69
Pivot joint, 14

Qualities of movement, 22, 24, 32, 33, 35, 36

Rallies, 87
Recording, 63
Relationships, 2, 5, 35–40, 49
Relaxation, 15, 19, 33, 41, 44, 53, 54
Resilience, 8, 11
Respiration, 18–19
Rhythm, 33, 34, 43, 45, 73, 75–76
Rising and sinking, 36, 38

Sensitivity, xiv, 32, 33, 46, 48
Shoulder girdle, 10
Simultaneous movements, 26
Skeleton, 6, 7
Slimming, 18
Small apparatus, 47, 49, 50, 60
  balls, 80–81
  clubs, 83–84
  hoops, 82–83
  materials, 84–85
Social value—*see* companionship
Sound accompaniment, 46–48
Space, 26–31
Space (effort), 33, 40
Spine, 8, 9, 20
Stillness, 25, 43
Strengthening movements, 11, 19, 42, 43–53
Successive movements, 26
Symmetry, 25, 31

Table plane, 30
Tactile stimuli, 80
Tape recordings, 79
Teacher—qualities, 4, 5, 70–71
  skills, 5, 48
  responsibilities, 5, 53, 58
Teaching methods, 43, 56, 67, 68
Tension, xiii, 4, 16, 17, 35, 44, 54
Theme, 45, 55, 58
Time, 33, 49
Turning, 24–25
Twisting, 8, 25

Weight (effort), 33, 39
Weight transference, 24
Wheel plane, 31